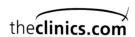
theclinics.com

CARDIOLOGY CLINICS

Heart Failure, Part I

GUEST EDITORS
James B. Young, MD
Jagat Narula, MD, PhD

CONSULTING EDITOR
Michael H. Crawford, MD

November 2007 • Volume 25 • Number 4

SAUNDERS

An Imprint of Elsevier, Inc.
PHILADELPHIA   LONDON   TORONTO   MONTREAL   SYDNEY   TOKYO

W.B. SAUNDERS COMPANY
A Division of Elsevier Inc.

Elsevier Inc. • 1600 John F. Kennedy Blvd., Suite 1800 • Philadelphia, Pennsylvania 19103-2899

http://www.theclinics.com

CARDIOLOGY CLINICS
November 2007
Editor: Barbara Cohen-Kligerman

Volume 25, Number 4
ISSN 0733-8651
ISBN-13: 978-1-4160-5043-8
ISBN-10: 1-4160-5043-4

Cardiology Clinics (ISSN 0733-8651) is published quarterly by Elsevier Inc., 360 Park Avenue South, New York, NY 10010-1710. Months of issue are February, May, August, and November. Business and editorial Offices: 1600 John F. Kennedy Blvd., Suite 1800, Philadelphia, PA 19103-2899. Customer Service Office: 6277 Sea Harbor Drive, Orlando, FL 32887-4800. Periodicals postage paid at New York, NY, and additional mailing offices. Subscription prices are $226.00 per year for US individuals, $344.00 per year for US institutions, $113.00 per year for US students and residents, $276.00 per year for Canadian individuals, $418.00 per year for Canadian institutions, $301.00 per year for international individuals, $418.00 per year for international institutions and $150.00 per year for Canadian and foreign students/residents. To receive student/resident rate, orders must be accompanied by name of affiliated institution, data of term, and the *signature* of program/residency coordinator on institution letterhead. Orders will be billed at individual rate until proof of status is received. Foreign air speed delivery is included in all *Clinics* subscription prices. All prices are subject to change without notice. POSTMASTER: Send address changes to *Cardiology Clinics*, Elsevier Periodicals Customer Service, 6277 Sea Harbor Drive, Orlando, FL 32887-4800. **Customer Service: 1-800-654-2452 (US). From outside of the US, call 1-407-345-1000.**

Cardiology Clinics is also published in Spanish by McGraw-Hill Interamericana Editores S. A., P.O. Box 5-237, 06500, Mexico D. F., Mexico; in Portuguese by Reichmann and Alfonso Editores Rio de Janeiro, Brazil; and in Greek by Dimitrios P. Lagos, 8 Pondon Street, GR115-28 Ilissia, Greece.

Cardiology Clinics is covered in *Index Medicus, Excerpta Medica, The Cumulative Index to Nursing and Allied Health Literature* (INAHL).

Printed in the United States of America.

CONSULTING EDITOR

MICHAEL H. CRAWFORD, MD, Professor of Medicine, University of California San Francisco; Lucie Stern Chair in Cardiology, and Interim Chief of Cardiology, University of California San Francisco Medical Center, San Francisco, California

GUEST EDITORS

JAMES B. YOUNG, MD, Chairman and Professor, Department of Medicine, Lerner College of Medicine; and George and Linda Kaufman Chair, Cleveland Clinic Foundation, Case Western Reserve University, Cleveland, Ohio

JAGAT NARULA, MD, PhD, Professor of Medicine, Chief, Division of Cardiology, University of California, Irvine School of Medicine, Orange, California

CONTRIBUTORS

RAGAVENDRA R. BALIGA, MD, MBA, FRCP, FACC, Director of Cardiovascular Medicine, University Hospitals East, Clinical Professor of Internal Medicine, The Ohio State University, Columbus, Ohio

DAVID S.H. BELL, MB, FACP, FACE, Adjunct Clinical Professor, University of Alabama Medical School, Birmingham, Alabama

SUSAN C. BROZENA, MD, Associate Professor of Medicine, Heart Failure/Transplant program, Cardiovascular Division, Department of Medicine, Hospital of the University of Pennsylvania, Philadelphia, Pennsylvania

DAVID A. CESARIO, MD, PhD, Assistant Clinical Professor of Medicine, Division of Cardiology, David Geffen School of Medicine at UCLA, Los Angeles, California

G. WILLIAM DEC, MD, Roman DeSanctis Professor of Medicine, Chief Cardiology, Cardiology Division, Massachusetts General Hospital, Boston, Massachusetts

ANITA DESWAL, MD, MPH, Winters Center for Heart Failure Research, Department of Medicine, Section of Cardiology, Michael E. DeBakey Veterans Affairs Medical Center, Houston, Texas

O.H. FRAZIER, MD, Director, Cardiopulmonary Transplant Service, Texas Heart Institute at St. Luke's Episcopal Hospital, Houston, Texas

LEON P. JACOB, MD, Surgery Fellow, Cardiopulmonary Transplant Service, Texas Heart Institute at St. Luke's Episcopal Hospital, Houston, Texas

MARIELL JESSUP, MD, Professor of Medicine, Heart Failure/Transplant program, Cardiovascular Division, Department of Medicine, Hospital of the University of Pennsylvania, Philadelphia, Pennsylvania

CARL V. LEIER, MD, The James W. Overstreet Professor of Medicine and Pharmacology, Division of Cardiovascular Disease, College of Medicine and Public Health, The Ohio State University, Columbus, Ohio

DOUGLAS L. MANN, MD, Winters Center for Heart Failure Research, Department of Medicine, Section of Cardiology, Michael E. DeBakey Veterans Affairs Medical Center, Baylor College of Medicine, Houston, Texas

KUMUDHA RAMASUBBU, MD, Winters Center for Heart Failure Research, Department of Medicine, Section of Cardiology, Michael E. DeBakey Veterans Affairs Medical Center, Baylor College of Medicine, Houston, Texas

WILLEM J. REMME, MD, PhD, Professor of Medicine, Sticares Cardiovascular Research Institute, Rhoon, The Netherlands

W.H. WILSON TANG, MD, FACC, FAHA, Assistant Professor of Medicine, Cleveland Clinic Lerner College of Medicine of Case Western Reserve University, Section of Heart Failure and Cardiac Transplantation Medicine, Department of Cardiovascular Medicine, Cleveland Clinic, Cleveland, Ohio

JONATHAN W. TURNER, MD, Medical Resident, David Geffen School of Medicine at UCLA, Los Angeles, California

RAMACHANDRAN S. VASAN, MD, National Heart, Lung and Blood Institute's Framingham Heart Study, Framingham, Massachusetts; and Cardiology section and Preventive Medicine, Department of Medicine, Boston University School of Medicine, Boston, Massachusetts

RAGHAVA S. VELAGALETI, MD, MPH, National Heart, Lung and Blood Institute's Framingham Heart Study, Framingham, Massachusetts

CONTENTS

> Hypertension and coronary disease are major risk factors for the incidence and progression of heart failure. These two risk factors frequently coexist, and have additive and synergistic effects that promote both left ventricular remodeling and heart failure in the general population. The relative contributions of these two risk factors to heart failure burden in the community may vary based on age, gender, and race. In general, attribution of heart failure in the community to solely one of these two risk factors is inappropriate. Prevention of both hypertension and coronary disease is important for preventing heart failure in the twenty-first century.

> The development of clinical or practice guidelines is thought to be a successful strategy for improving quality of care. Accordingly, many professional organizations, societies, institutions of health care or policy, and even countries have published practice guidelines on a variety of topics, including heart failure.

> If the recommendations of Joint National Committee 7 are implemented, the incidence of heart failure should continue to decline. These recommendations are designed not only to reduce the incidence of heart failure but also prevent other target end-organ damage and reduce overall cardiovascular morbidity and mortality. The emphasis of these recommendations is to reduce systolic blood pressure, because the risk of mortality caused by heart disease and stroke doubles for every 20-mm Hg increase in systolic

blood pressure. Practitioners are encouraged to use a combination of lifestyle changes and pharmacotherapy to achieve systolic blood pressure goals and consider the use of thiazide diuretics as first-line therapy to achieve the ultimate goal of reducing end-organ damage.

focused on agents that block the RAS. More recently, the role of angiotensin receptor blockers (ARBs) in heart failure therapy has been better defined. This article examines the rationale and role of ARBs in the treatment of patients with heart failure on the basis of evidence from clinical trials.

FORTHCOMING ISSUES

RECENT ISSUES

ELSEVIER
SAUNDERS

Cardiol Clin 25 (2007) ix

CARDIOLOGY
CLINICS

Foreword

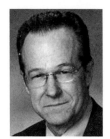

Michael H. Crawford, MD
Consulting Editor

The last issue of *Cardiology Clinics* devoted to heart failure was published in 2001, and the guest editor was Dr. Young. Since then, major advances have been made in our understanding of heart failure, and new treatment options are now available. I was delighted, therefore, when Dr. Young teamed up with Dr. Narula to guest edit two issues devoted to this topic. Heart failure mortality has decreased significantly in the last 10 years mainly because of advances in therapy. It is important to know about these advances so your patients can benefit. Despite the decrease in mortality, the prevalence of heart failure is increasing. The future of heart failure is prevention. Drs. Young and Narula launch this issue with a discussion of the new direction in heart failure prevention.

The first section of this issue starts with a description of the scope of the heart failure problem. Unfortunately, many have been confused by different heart failure management guidelines from professional organizations. These are discussed, as is the relevance of the Joint National Committee and the American Diabetes Association guidelines to heart failure prevention and treatment.

The second section of this issue updates the management of advanced and decompensated heart failure. Who needs hemodynamic monitoring? What about intravenous natriuretic peptides and positive inotropes? Finally, mechanical circulatory support is discussed. I have been impressed

that these new devices are now saving lives with low risk to the patient. We have come a long way since the intraaortic balloon pump.

The last section of this issue covers the therapy for chronic heart failure. Several new drugs that affect the renin-angiotensin-aldosterone system are described. What to start first, beta-blockers or angiotensin-reducing or -blocking agents, is discussed. Finally, the use of implantable cardioverter defibrillators and biventricular pacing is detailed. The increased use of these valuable electronic devices is creating a natural synergy between heart failure specialists and electrophysiologists. Add cardiac transplant surgeons and those who put in mechanical circulatory support devices and you have the new team that manages advanced heart failure in referral centers. In many centers such a team has its own cost center independent of traditional academic departments. Welcome to the new world of heart failure management.

Michael H. Crawford, MD
Division of Cardiology
Department of Medicine
University of California
San Francisco Medical Center
505 Parnassus Avenue, Box 0124
San Francisco, CA 94143-0124, USA

E-mail address: crawfordm@medicine.ucsf.edu

Preface
Prevention Should Take Center Stage

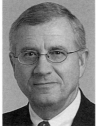 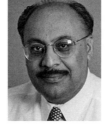

James B. Young, MD   Jagat Narula, MD, PhD
Guest Editors

The trends of the population pool of any infirmity depend upon the number of patients added to and removed from the pool in a unit of time. The demographics of heart failure (HF) have witnessed marked changes in the last 50 years. HF mortality has declined by almost one half in the last 10 years, and HF as a discharge diagnosis has increased by threefold in the last 30 years. A progressive increase is expected in the older population in America in the coming years, with a proportional increase in the number of patients who have HF. Improvements in the management of acute coronary syndromes have inflated the number of surviving patients, particularly male patients, who have residual systolic dysfunction. Whereas all preceding factors have added to the pool size, extensive use of antihypertensive therapy has lowered the burden of HF, particularly in women. It is evident that the burden of HF will not be eliminated by an improvement in the survival of patients who are already affected; instead, a drastic reduction in the incidence of HF is required to prevent an increase in the HF burden.

In 2005, the American College of Cardiology/ American Heart Association (ACC/AHA) proposed a new staging classification for HF. ACC/ AHA guidelines for the diagnosis and management of HF identify four stages, A through D [1]. These guidelines recognize the risk factors and structural prerequisites for the development of HF. This classification proposes that patients advance to higher stages as part of the natural history of HF unless progression is slowed or stopped. It is suggested that intervention be initiated before significant left ventricular (LV) dysfunction or symptoms occur.

Stage A patients are at high risk for developing heart failure but do not yet have structural heart disease or symptoms of heart failure. This stage includes patients who have hypertension, diabetes, hyperlipidemia, obesity, metabolic syndrome, and atherosclerotic disease. When first proposed, this category was highly controversial, because critics questioned the inclusion of a group of individuals who, by definition, do not have a traditional "congestive heart failure" syndrome. This argument was successfully countered as the profession became more aware that even in some asymptomatic individuals (eg, those who have grossly normal heart structure and hypertension) there is an insidious and progressive failure of myocyte molecular biodynamics that in more normal circumstances would maintain normal homeostasis. This condition came to be recognized as cardiac

0733-8651/07/$ - see front matter © 2007 Elsevier Inc. All rights reserved.
doi:10.1016/j.ccl.2007.10.002

cardiology.theclinics.com

"failure" of a sort. Obviously, the management of these individuals includes blood pressure control; treatment of dyslipidemia, diabetes, and the metabolic syndrome; and lifestyle changes such as smoking cessation and exercise.

Patients who are diagnosed as having structural myocardial disease but who have never experienced symptoms of heart failure are classified as stage B. Included among these patients are those who have LV remodeling manifested by LV hypertrophy, those who have had myocardial infarction, and those who have asymptomatic valvular heart disease. The management of these patients includes beta-blockers, angiotensin-converting enzyme inhibitors (ACE-I), and, in selected cases, defibrillators. Stage C patients are those who have known heart failure with current or prior symptoms. The management of these patients includes diuretics, ACE-I, beta-blockers, aldosterone receptor blockers, diuretics, digoxin, hydralazine/nitrate, biventricular pacemakers, and defibrillators. Stage D patients include those who have advanced symptoms after optimal medical care. The management of these patients includes inotropes, cardiac transplantation, mechanical circulatory devices, specialized surgical techniques, and palliative care.

This staging system considers HF to be similar to coronary artery disease, in that it has established risk factors and structural prerequisites and recognizes that the development of HF has asymptomatic and symptomatic phases. Also, each stage is targeted with specific therapies, many of which are known to reduce the morbidity and mortality of HF. This staging system is similar to the staging system for pre-cancer and cancer, in which patients can either remain stable, without disease progression, or advance from one stage to the next unless this progression is slowed or stopped by therapy.

The progression of HF mandates that an all-out effort be made to prevent its development in the first place, and the best time to intervene would be before or at pre-HF stage A. Optimal management of these patients requires adherence to various guidelines targeted at control of risk factors, such as the Adult Treatment Panel III goals for plasma LDL and HDL [2,3] and the Joint National Committee on Prevention, Detection, Evaluation, and Treatment of High Blood Pressure goals for systolic and diastolic blood pressure [4,5], the ACC/AHA goals for metabolic syndrome and the American Diabetes Association recommendations for diabetes mellitus. Hypertension and myocardial infarction together account for approximately three fourths of the population-attributable risk of HF [6], and both are, by and large, preventable with currently known and available strategies (Fig. 1) [7].

The importance of elevated blood pressure is demonstrated by the twofold increase in risk of HF among those who have systolic blood pressure (BP) levels above 160 mm Hg and diastolic BP levels above 90 mm Hg compared with those who have both systolic BP levels below 140 mm Hg and diastolic BP levels below 90 mm Hg. This risk is

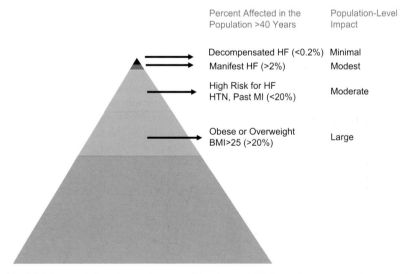

Fig. 1. Pyramid of HF in population. (*Data from* Yusuf S, Pitt B. A lifetime of prevention: the case of heart failure. Circulation 2002;106:2997–8.)

likely to be continuous, so even lower rates of HF can be expected among those who have systolic BP levels below 120 mm Hg. A 5–mm Hg drop in a population's systolic BP could, by itself, reduce the age-specific rates of HF by about one fourth. In persons who have hypertension (prevalence, $\sim$ 20%), a 10–mm Hg reduction in systolic BP has been shown to reduce the incidence of HF by 50%. Therefore, a combined strategy of hypertension therapy along with lifestyle modifications to lower the mean BP should reduce age-specific rates of HF in the population by more than one third and possibly by as much as one half.

The second major antecedent cause of HF is myocardial infarction. The risk of myocardial infarction can be reduced by modification of classic risk factors (eg, lowering LDL cholesterol, increasing HDL [8], lowering BP). These risk factors can be modified favorably through lifestyle changes, including reduction of weight and tobacco cessation efforts. The importance of obesity in causing HF has been shown by the Framingham Heart Study [9]. Obesity is a proximate risk factor for HF and may exert its influence both directly and indirectly, by promoting hypertension, diabetes, dyslipidemia, metabolic syndrome, and atherosclerosis. Therefore, efforts to prevent obesity are likely to have an impact on a number of manifestations of cardiovascular disease, including HF. Treatment of hypertension reduces the incidence of HF by approximately 50%, even among very elderly patients. Statins reduce the incidence of HF by approximately 20% among patients who have dyslipidemia and coronary artery disease [10]. ACE inhibitors reduce incidence of HF by 37% among patients who have reduced LV systolic function and by 23% among patients who have coronary artery disease and normal systolic function [10]. Observational studies have reported a lower incidence of HF among diabetics who have better glycemic control [10].

The ACC/AHA has set the stage for prevention of heart failure by including pre-HF in its staging categories. For preventive strategies to be fully effective against HF, they must be implemented throughout the lifetime of an individual. It is high time for prevention of HF to take center stage.

James B. Young, MD
Cleveland Clinic Foundation, Cleveland, OH

E-mail address: youngj@ccf.org

Jagat Narula, MD, PhD
University of California, Irvine, CA

E-mail address: Narula@uci.edu

References

[1] Hunt SA, Abraham WT, Chin MH, et al. ACC/AHA 2005 Guideline. Update for the diagnosis and management of chronic heart failure in the adult: a report of the American College of Cardiology/American Heart Association Task Force on Practice Guidelines (Writing Committee to Update the 2001 Guidelines for the Evaluation and Management of Heart Failure): developed in collaboration with the American College of Chest Physicians and the International Society for Heart and Lung Transplantation: endorsed by the Heart Rhythm Society. Circulation 2005; 112(12):e154–235.

[2] Executive summary of the third report of the National Cholesterol Education Program (NCEP) Expert Panel on Detection, Evaluation, and Treatment of High Blood Cholesterol in Adults (Adult Treatment Panel III). JAMA 2001;285(19): 2486–97.

[3] Third report of the National Cholesterol Education Program (NCEP) Expert Panel on Detection, Evaluation, and Treatment of High Blood Cholesterol in Adults (Adult Treatment Panel III) final report. Circulation 2002;106(25):3143–421.

[4] Chobanian AV, Bakris GL, Black HR, et al. The seventh report of the Joint National Committee on Prevention, Detection, Evaluation, and Treatment of High Blood Pressure: the JNC 7 report. JAMA 2003;289(19):2560–7252.

[5] Fagard RH, Staessen JA, Thijs L, et al. On-treatment diastolic blood pressure and prognosis in systolic hypertension. Arch Intern Med 2007;167(17): 1884–91.

[6] Lloyd-Jones DM, Larson MG, Leip EP, et al. Lifetime risk for developing congestive heart failure: the Framingham Heart Study. Circulation 2002; 106(24):3068–72.

[7] Yusuf S, Pitt B. A lifetime of prevention: the case of heart failure. Circulation 2002;106(24):2997–8.

[8] Barter P, Gotto AM, LaRosa JC, et al. HDL cholesterol, very low levels of LDL cholesterol, and cardiovascular events. N Engl J Med 2007;357(13): 1301–10.

[9] Kenchaiah S, Evans JC, Levy D, et al. Obesity and the risk of heart failure. N Engl J Med 2002;347(5): 305–13.

[10] Baker DW. Prevention of heart failure. J Card Fail 2002;8(5):333–46.

Heart Failure in the Twenty-First Century: Is it a Coronary Artery Disease or Hypertension Problem?

Raghava S. Velagaleti, MD, MPH[a], Ramachandran S. Vasan, MD[a,b,*]

[a]Framingham Heart Study, Framingham, MA, USA
[b]Boston University School of Medicine, Boston, MA, USA

Heart failure is the third most prevalent cardiovascular disease in the United States. An estimated 5 million people in the United States have heart failure, and the prevalence of the condition will increase to 10 million by 2040, according to predictions [1–3]. The prevalence of heart failure increases with age from less than 1% in the 20- to 39-year-old age group to over 20% in people age 80 years or older [4]. The lifetime risk of developing heart failure is estimated at about 20% in both men and women [4]. Even without antecedent coronary artery disease (CAD), the lifetime risk of developing heart failure at age 40 is estimated at 11.4% for men and 15.4% for women [4]. In addition to people with overt heart failure, an estimated 74 million people are living with risk factors for heart failure (ie, are in stage A of heart failure) [2,3]. More than 500,000 new cases of heart failure are diagnosed each year, and this incidence is expected to rise to 772,000 new cases per year by 2040 [5]. Heart failure also accounts for 12 million to 15 million office visits and 6.5 million days of hospital stay each year [6]. The number of hospitalizations for heart failure has risen to over a million per year over the past decade. The estimated economic burden of caring for patients with overt heart failure is $27 billion to $38 billion, with 10% of this amount being spent on drugs alone [2,6].

As noted, heart failure is also characterized by substantial morbidity and mortality. Nearly 50,000 people die annually of heart failure [3]. Despite major advances in treatment, the prognosis after a diagnosis of heart failure is still dire and comparable to that of several forms of cancer [7]. Even though the rate of fatalities per cases associated with heart failure has been declining [8], the crude number of deaths attributed to the condition has been increasing, primarily because of increasing prevalence of the condition. The aging of the population and improved survival and "salvage" of patients with myocardial infarction (with subsequent progression to pump failure) are believed to be some factors contributing to the growing burden of heart failure.

Several epidemiological investigations have identified risk factors for heart failure [9]. Increasing age, hypertension, coronary artery disease, diabetes, obesity, valvular heart disease, and the metabolic syndrome are key risk factors for heart failure [9,10]. In recent years, many genetic risk factors have also been identified [11]. The relative contribution of risk factors to the occurrence of heart failure in the community may be changing over time. Data from the Framingham Heart Study demonstrate that, from the 1950s onwards, the contribution of valvular disease to the burden of heart failure has steadily declined, whereas the role of myocardial infarction has increased substantially [4,8].

Given the sizeable public health burden posed by heart failure, and limited health care

This work was supported by NO1-HC-25195, K24 HL 04334 (RSV), from the National Heart, Lung and Blood Institute.

* Corresponding author. Framingham Heart Study, 73 Mount Wayte Avenue, Suite 2 Framingham, MA 01702-5803.

E-mail address: vasan@bu.edu (R.S. Vasan).

resources, it is critical to identify the primary "drivers" of this problem. Identification of the key risk factors in order of their relative importance will help guide health policy and resource allocation, and aid in the formulation of efficient preventive and therapeutic approaches targeting heart failure. Also, a majority of people with the "pre–heart-failure" phenotype (stages A and B) and overt heart failure are "cared for" by primary care physicians, underscoring the importance of providing clear guidance on risk factors that warrant a primary focus to prevent the future burden of heart failure. Given that hypertension and CAD are the major modifiable risk factors for heart failure [12,13], this article appraises the relative contributions of these two conditions to heart failure burden, providing context for this debate.

Is heart failure primarily a problem of coronary artery disease?

Biological plausibility and mechanistic insights

Coronary atherosclerosis is the critical determinant of the clinical manifestations of CAD. The role of myocardial infarction as a major antecedent of heart failure has been established by several studies [9,14–16]. Clinically silent coronary disease is widely prevalent both in the general population and in heart failure patients, as evidenced by coronary plaques found both in children and young adults in autopsy series [17] and in angiographic studies of healthy heart-transplant donors [18]. In addition to epicardial disease, microvascular coronary disease is also both widespread and often under-recognized [19]. These data suggest that CAD (epicardial or microvascular; clinically overt or silent) can lead to decreased perfusion of the myocardium (both acutely and chronically), thereby predisposing to myocardial damage with its sequel of decreased myocardial function.

CAD can lead to heart failure by several mechanisms. Four such mechanisms are associated with acute myocardial infarction, which frequently leads to permanent death of cardiac muscle. One of these is diastolic dysfunction. This occurs because the infarcted segment is akinetic/dyskinetic, thus leading to inadequate relaxation in diastole and impaired contraction in systole. Diastolic dysfunction is present early in myocardial infarction, and may be related to the development of in-hospital heart failure and death [20]. The impairment of ventricular function after MI is usually improved with the early restoration of coronary blood flow in the culprit vessel, with either thrombolysis, angioplasty or with bypass surgery [21,22]. A second mechanism by which acute myocardial infarction can lead to heart failure is related to the scar formation in the area where the infarct heals. Here an aneurysm may form, which can further impair contractile performance and relaxation. A third mechanism by which myocardial infarction can result in heart failure is the dyssynchronous contraction of the infarcted segment, which can decrease the efficiency of pump function. A fourth mechanism for heart failure occurs in the context of rupture of the mitral or submitral apparatus as a result of ischemic injury (papillary muscle rupture or flail leaflet), which can result in acute severe mitral regurgitation and acute onset of heart failure [23,24].

Changes in the ventricle away from the site of myocardial insult or injury can also contribute to heart failure risk. Whereas the initial myocardial injury and scarring can result in regional dysfunction at the site of injury, subsequent remodeling of the ventricle can occur in myocardial segments remote from the site of infarction. Such regional remodeling frequently results in a distortion of ventricular structure and geometry, and can contribute to a further decline in ventricular function [25]. Ventricular dilatation can promote annular dilation, with consequent mitral regurgitation, which can predispose to heart failure.

Chronic dysfunction of the myocardium resulting from hypoperfusion, hibernation, or both hypoperfusion and hibernation may also enhance the risk of heart failure [26,27]. Patients with both epicardial and endocardial CAD may have chronic hypoperfusion, which leads to increased myocardial stiffness secondary to chronic inflammation and fibrosis. Patients with episodic decreases in coronary perfusion may demonstrate impairment of myocardial function for hours or days (myocardial stunning) [28]. Studies with positron emission tomography [29] and single photon emission computed tomography [30] demonstrate decreased blood flow and glucose uptake in myocardial regions that can simultaneously be shown to have decreased systolic function. Ventricular diastolic function has been shown to be decreased in both experimental [31] and clinical ischemia [32]. Also, the coronary vasodilator reserve decreases in proportion to degree of luminal stenosis of the coronary arteries [33,34]. Consequently, areas of the myocardium with normal blood flow at rest may have reduced myocardial blood flow during exercise, and may demonstrate reduced glucose metabolism on positron emission tomography during exercise, with a concomitant decrease in ventricular function.

Epidemiological studies identifying coronary artery disease as a major contributor to heart failure burden

Some reports have demonstrated that epicardial CAD is an etiological factor in a third of patients with heart failure [35]. Across several studies, CAD has been reported to account for 23% to73% of the heart failure in the patients evaluated. Some investigators have argued that the most common cause of heart failure is CAD [36]. Framingham data indicate a differential contribution of CAD to heart failure burden in men versus women. The population attributable risk (PAR) for heart failure associated with CAD is 39% in men, but only 18% in women [37]. In heart failure series that focused on patients with a reduced left ventricular ejection fraction, CAD is usually the major cause [35]. Autopsy series indicate that a third of patients with heart failure have prevalent but undetected major coronary artery disease [38]. Thus, even in heart failure patients classified clinically as "nonischemic cardiomyopathy," up to a fourth may have evidence of CAD at autopsy [39]. Also, ischemic changes have been demonstrated on endomyocardial biopsies [40] in such patients. Indeed, such patients with so-called "nonischemic cardiomyopathy" may develop clinical ischemic events on subsequent follow-up, an observation that suggests that coronary disease may not be just a "bystander" in these patients [41]. The frequent presence if microvascular disease detected with positron emission tomography scanning [42] or with Doppler flow velocimetry [43] in response to stress in such patients further incriminates CAD as a potential contributor to the ventricular dysfunction.

The presence of underlying CAD also contributes to the morbidity and mortality of patients with heart failure [44]. Angiographic evidence of CAD has been shown to be a marker of a worse prognosis in heart failure patients [45], with the mortality risk being increased by 250% in some reports [46].

In summary, perfusion abnormalities are likely present in the vast majority of patients with heart failure (including those categorized as "nonischemic"), rendering coronary disease as the predominant determinant of heart failure.

Evidence linking CAD to heart failure from clinical trials

Clinical trials of post–myocardial-infarction patients suggest that prompt and appropriately targeted therapy can lower the risk of developing ventricular dysfunction and overt heart failure after ischemic injury, thereby further suggesting a causal relationship between CAD and heart failure [47–49]. In the last decade, several large trials of myocardial infarction patients have evaluated the incidence of new-onset heart failure as an endpoint (in addition to decrease in death, nonfatal myocardial infarction, and need for revascularization), and have shown a reduction in heart failure incidence with several treatment strategies [50–52]. It is also well established that acute coronary events can precipitate the decompensation of patients with chronic compensated heart failure. It has been argued that the benefit of angiotensin-converting enzyme (ACE) inhibitors and beta-blockers in heart failure trials lags behind the immediate hemodynamic improvement seen with these agents, raising the possibility that the accrual of benefits over time may be due to amelioration of coronary disease in some patients [36]. Coronary revascularization in selected patients ameliorates diastolic function abnormalities, reduces morbidity and mortality [53–56], and may improve systolic function [57], likely by "recruitment" of hibernating myocardium.

In summary, extensive data from a basic science perspective, epidemiological studies, and clinical trials suggest that CAD is a principal contributor to heart failure burden. As more and more "high-risk" patients survive after CAD events because of accruing improvements in management strategies, it is conceivable that the burden of heart failure due to CAD may increase in the future. Indeed CAD may be the key risk factor for heart failure in the new millennium.

Is heart failure primarily a hypertension problem?

Biological plausibility and mechanistic insights

Systemic blood pressure is determined by peripheral vascular resistance and conduit artery stiffness. The myocardium has to pump blood against the afterload posed by the resistance of peripheral vasculature and the stiffness of the large and medium-sized arteries. An elevated blood pressure places greater hemodynamic burden on the myocardium.

Elevated blood pressure leads to a compensatory increase in myocardial muscle mass to maintain normal cardiac output [58,59]. In both hypertensive and prehypertensive states, there is slow but steady hypertrophy of the left ventricle [60,61]. This is associated initially with myocardial stiffness and a decreased ability to relax and fill, initially during exercise and subsequently at rest [62–65]. Ventricular diastolic dysfunction due to high blood pressure is an important contributor to the development of overt heart failure. Indeed, the prognosis of heart failure patients has been related to ventricular filling abnormalities regardless of ventricular ejection fraction [66]. In addition, left ventricular mass increases disproportionately in hypertension relative to the ability of the microvasculature [67] to perfuse the hypertrophied myocardium both at rest and during exercise, thereby proving to be a "setup" for chronic subendocardial hypoperfusion.

The progression from chronic hypertension to structural ventricular changes, and then to asymptomatic systolic and diastolic ventricular dysfunction is well established by natural history investigations from longitudinal epidemiological cohort studies, such as the Framingham Heart Study [37]. Acute hypertensive crises can also cause heart failure. Experimental data as well as human studies have also demonstrated that sudden acute increases in blood pressure (such as in hypertensive emergencies) can lead to acute left ventricular strain and manifest as hypertensive heart failure [68]. Also, an acute elevation of blood pressure is a common precipitating cause for the decompensation of a patient with compensated chronic heart failure [69]. Thus, both chronic and acute hypertension have been linked to the risk of heart failure.

Epidemiological studies identifying hypertension as a major contributor to heart failure burden

From an epidemiological perspective, hypertension is the most prevalent cardiovascular risk factor. An estimated 72 million Americans have high blood pressure, with millions more having a "prehypertensive" state. Investigators have demonstrated that prehypertension also elevates the risk of developing heart disease [70].

Hypertension is an antecedent of the vast majority of individuals with heart failure in the community, as suggested by data from the Framingham Study [37]. The PAR for heart failure associated with hypertension was 39% in men and 59% in women in a report from the Framingham Study [37]. Although the PAR for hypertension has decreased over the last five decades, the prevalence of hypertension is increasing and a substantial proportion of individuals with hypertension do not have their blood pressure controlled to recommended levels [71]. Also, hypertension is frequently accompanied by metabolic risk factors and obesity, which themselves increase the risk of heart failure. With the rising societal burden of obesity and the metabolic syndrome [72], it is conceivable that, without better rates of control of cardiovascular risk factors (including elevated blood pressure), the contribution of hypertension and prehypertension to ventricular remodeling and heart failure in the community may increase in this millennium.

Evidence from clinical trials linking hypertension to heart failure

A number of clinical trials demonstrate the benefit of treating hypertension in the prevention and treatment of heart failure [73–75]. Primary prevention trials demonstrate up to a 50% reduction in the incidence of heart failure in patients with hypertension who are treated with blood pressure lowering agents [76]. In patients with established cardiovascular disease, treating blood pressure to targets advocated by the Joint National Committee on Prevention, Detection, Evaluation, and Treatment of High Blood Pressure reduced further incidence of recurrent events and also the progression to heart failure [77]. In patients with left ventricular systolic dysfunction [78] or left ventricular hypertrophy, control of blood pressure prevents or retards ventricular remodeling and decreases the incidence of overt heart failure [79]. In patients with established heart failure, further decreases of blood pressure with therapy may lower the mortality rate, slow the progression of disease, reduce the number of hospitalizations and exacerbations, and enhance quality of life and functional capacity [14].

The pivotal role of high blood pressure in the pathophysiology of heart failure may be inferred by the profound benefits of afterload reducing agents in improving clinical outcomes in patients, relative to a lesser magnitude of benefit achieved by using inotropic agents. ACE inhibitors, angiotensin receptor blockers, hydralazine (in combination with nitroglycerine), and dihydro-pyridine calcium channel blockers all reduce morbidity and mortality in heart failure, as opposed to a lack of survival benefits with the use of diuretics, digoxin, phosphodiesterase inhibitors, and inotropes [2]. Thus, clinical data support the contention that higher systemic blood pressure is a dominant determinant of heart failure risk.

Not only is chronic hypertension a problem, but acute elevations in blood pressure can also precipitate episodes of heart failure [68]. Also, recurrent catecholamine surges, as seen in sleep apnea and the blunting of the nocturnal declines in blood pressure, have been linked to heart failure risk [80]. It is also important to recall that hypertension is a common condition. As such, the PAR associated with a common condition is likely to be higher, even if the relative risk of heart failure is higher for CAD (or myocardial infarction).

In summary, considerable evidence from experimental and clinical studies and epidemiological investigations indicate the critical role of hypertension in the pathogenesis of heart failure. The lifetime risk of hypertension is estimated to be 90% [81]. Thus, a compelling argument can be made that hypertension may be a key contributor to heart failure risk in the new millennium. Clearly, if we are able to prevent hypertension and control blood pressure in those with established hypertension, the risks associated with hypertension may diminish in this millennium.

Discussion: Is this a reasonable debate?

Thus, persuasive arguments can be made to substantiate the claims that either CAD or hypertension may be key etiological risk factors for heart failure in the new millennium. But it is worth pondering if this is, in reality, a reasonable debate. Several issues have to be considered to ascertain the primacy of one risk factor over others. Hypertension and CAD frequently coexist. The two conditions also interact synergistically as risk factors for heart failure (see below). Also, the relative impact of the two conditions may differ according to age, gender, race, and other factors. It is well established that blacks face a higher burden of blood-pressure–related conditions, including heart failure, compared with whites in whom CAD is more often a culprit [3,37]. Lastly, as outlined below, there can be the ascertainment bias in the adjudication of a particular risk factor as the primary etiological factor for heart failure.

High blood pressure is a powerful risk factor for CAD, with a continuous gradient of risk that starts at levels below what is recognized as hypertension [82,83]. Hypertension is also a risk factor for left ventricular hypertrophy, which itself has been shown to be associated with a two- to fivefold increase in myocardial infarction on long-term follow-up [76]. Also, hypertension can contribute to ischemia by increasing myocardial oxygen demand (by increased workload imposed on the heart), in the setting of diminished subendocardial blood supply in concentric hypertrophy [84]. Experimental data demonstrate that hypertrophied hearts demonstrate subendocardial ischemia during pacing-induced tachycardia and during exercise even in the absence of epicardial coronary disease [85,86]. In addition, hypertension can precipitate acute coronary syndromes via shear stress, which can contribute to the rupture of unstable plaques [87].

Widespread atherosclerosis has also been implicated in the pathogenesis of vascular stiffness and decreased vascular reactivity. Such atherosclerosis-related increased vascular stiffness and endothelial dysfunction may contribute to higher peripheral vascular resistance and blood pressure [88,89]. Also, renal artery atherosclerosis can lead to increased activation of the renin-angiotensin-aldosterone system (RAAS) pathway and cause hypertension. The impact of statins in effectively improving systemic [90] and coronary [91] vasoreactivity is consistent with the notion that atherosclerosis can be a cause, not just a consequence, of elevated blood pressure (though other pleiotropic effects of statins may also contribute to these observations).

In addition, a common set of biological pathways has been implicated in the pathogenesis of both hypertension and CAD. The most notable such pathway is the RAAS. The activation of RAAS is a major mechanism in the development and establishment of both primary and secondary hypertension [92]. Use of agents that block the RAAS with aldosterone antagonists (eg, eplerenone) or renin inhibition (eg, aliskiren) is a key antihypertensive management strategy. Activation of RAAS is also implicated in CAD. Biomarkers of RAAS activation (eg, plasma renin activity [93] and aldosterone levels [94]) correlate vascular function [95] and with cardiovascular outcomes [96]. Treatment with agents that interfere with the RAAS pathway (eg, ACE inhibitors, angiotensin receptor blockers, and eplerenone) reduce the risk of cardiovascular outcomes, thereby definitively establishing the pivotal role of this pathway. RAAS is also instrumental in the progression of heart failure. ACE inhibition and aldosterone antagonism are the most established strategies to control blood pressure, restore endothelial function, stop or reverse left ventricular hypertrophy, improve microcirculation, improve left ventricular function, and improve survival in hypertension, CAD, and heart failure. Thus, common underlying pathogenetic mechanisms preclude any attempts to simplify heart failure as a "one-major-factor–related" condition. A majority of heart failure patients have both CAD and hypertension, thus further rendering moot the discussion of which factor to "blame more."

Summary

Both hypertension and CAD are major risk factors for the onset and the progression of heart failure. They have additive and synergistic effects in the pathogenesis of the syndrome, and frequently coexist. With the aging of the population in developed countries and with onset of epidemiological transition of developing countries (to the stage of chronic degenerative diseases) [97], the prevalence of hypertension, CAD, and heart failure will likely rise worldwide over the next few decades. Fortunately, our understanding of these conditions and their treatments is robust, rendering this challenge as an opportunity to implement better preventive methods.

Obesity, atherogenic diet, sedentary lifestyle, and smoking underlie adult development of metabolic syndrome, vascular risk factors (including hypertension), and CAD. As Kannel [98] pointed out: "Overt heart failure is now better regarded as medical failure rather than indication for treatment." Thus future endeavors to reduce heart failure burden must include primordial prevention (the prevention of risk factors themselves), not just management of existing risk factors or established disease.

References

[1] Executive summary. HFSA 2006 Comprehensive Heart Failure Practice Guideline. J Card Fail 2006; 12(1):10–38.

[2] Hunt SA, Abraham WT, Chin MH, et al. ACC/AHA 2005 guideline update for the diagnosis and management of chronic heart failure in the adult: a report of the American College of Cardiology/American Heart Association Task Force on Practice Guidelines (Writing Committee to Update the 2001 Guidelines for the Evaluation and Management of Heart Failure): developed in collaboration with the American College of Chest Physicians and the International Society for Heart and Lung Transplantation: endorsed by the Heart Rhythm Society. Circulation 2005;112(12):e154–235.

[3] Rosamond W, Flegal K, Friday G, et al. Heart disease and stroke statistics—2007 update: a report from the American Heart Association Statistics Committee and Stroke Statistics Subcommittee. Circulation 2007;115(5):e69–171.

[4] Lloyd-Jones DM, Larson MG, Leip EP, et al. Lifetime risk for developing congestive heart failure: the Framingham Heart Study. Circulation 2002; 106(24):3068–72.

[5] Owan TE, Redfield MM. Epidemiology of diastolic heart failure. Prog Cardiovasc Dis 2005;47(5): 320–32.

[6] O'Connell JB, Bristow MR. Economic impact of heart failure in the United States: time for a different approach. J Heart Lung Transplant 1994;13(4): S107–12.

[7] Ho KK, Anderson KM, Kannel WB, et al. Survival after the onset of congestive heart failure in Framingham Heart Study subjects. Circulation 1993; 88(1):107–15.

[8] Levy D, Kenchaiah S, Larson MG, et al. Long-term trends in the incidence of and survival with heart failure. N Engl J Med 2002;347(18):1397–402.

[9] Kenchaiah S, Narula J, Vasan RS. Risk factors for heart failure. Med Clin North Am 2004;88(5): 1145–72.

[10] Kenchaiah S, Evans JC, Levy D, et al. Obesity and the risk of heart failure. N Engl J Med 2002;347(5): 305–13.

[11] Maron BJ, Towbin JA, Thiene G, et al. Contemporary definitions and classification of the cardiomyopathies: an American Heart Association Scientific Statement from the Council on Clinical Cardiology, Heart Failure and Transplantation Committee; Quality of Care and Outcomes Research and Functional Genomics and Translational Biology Interdisciplinary Working Groups; and Council on Epidemiology and Prevention. Circulation 2006; 113(14):1807–16.

[12] Gillum RF. Epidemiology of heart failure in the United States. Am Heart J 1993;126(4):1042–7.

[13] McKee PA, Castelli WP, McNamara PM, et al. The natural history of congestive heart failure: the Framingham study. N Engl J Med 1971;285(26): 1441–6.

[14] Packer M, Coats AJ, Fowler MB, et al. Effect of carvedilol on survival in severe chronic heart failure. N Engl J Med 2001;344(22):1651–8.

[15] Bourassa MG, Gurne O, Bangdiwala SI, et al. Natural history and patterns of current practice in heart failure. The Studies of Left Ventricular Dysfunction

(SOLVD) Investigators. J Am Coll Cardiol 1993; 22(4 Suppl A):14A–9A.

[16] Torp-Pedersen C, Moller M, Bloch-Thomsen PE, et al. Dofetilide in patients with congestive heart failure and left ventricular dysfunction. Danish Investigations of Arrhythmia and Mortality on Dofetilide Study Group. N Engl J Med 1999; 341(12):857–65.

[17] Kavey RE, Daniels SR, Lauer RM, et al. American Heart Association guidelines for primary prevention of atherosclerotic cardiovascular disease beginning in childhood. Circulation 2003;107(11):1562–6.

[18] Tuzcu EM, Kapadia SR, Tutar E, et al. High prevalence of coronary atherosclerosis in asymptomatic teenagers and young adults: evidence from intravascular ultrasound. Circulation 2001;103(22):2705–10.

[19] Mohri M, Takeshita A. Coronary microvascular disease in humans. Jpn Heart J 1999;40(2):97–108.

[20] Poulsen SH, Jensen SE, Egstrup K. Longitudinal changes and prognostic implications of left ventricular diastolic function in first acute myocardial infarction. Am Heart J 1999;137(5):910–8.

[21] Humphrey LS, Topol EJ, Rosenfeld GI, et al. Immediate enhancement of left ventricular relaxation by coronary artery bypass grafting: intraoperative assessment. Circulation 1988;77(4):886–96.

[22] Bonow RO, Vitale DF, Bacharach SL, et al. Asynchronous left ventricular regional function and impaired global diastolic filling in patients with coronary artery disease: reversal after coronary angioplasty. Circulation 1985;71(2):297–307.

[23] Hochman JS, Boland J, Sleeper LA, et al. Current spectrum of cardiogenic shock and effect of early revascularization on mortality. Results of an International Registry. SHOCK Registry Investigators. Circulation 1995;91(3):873–81.

[24] Lavie CJ, Gersh BJ. Mechanical and electrical complications of acute myocardial infarction. Mayo Clin Proc 1990;65(5):709–30.

[25] Sutton MG, Sharpe N. Left ventricular remodeling after myocardial infarction: pathophysiology and therapy. Circulation 2000;101(25):2981–8.

[26] Wijns W, Vatner SF, Camici PG. Hibernating myocardium. N Engl J Med 1998;339(3):173–81.

[27] Kloner RA, Przyklenk K. Hibernation and stunning of the myocardium. N Engl J Med 1991;325(26): 1877–9.

[28] Bolli R. Myocardial 'stunning' in man. Circulation 1992;86(6):1671–91.

[29] Auerbach MA, Schoder H, Hoh C, et al. Prevalence of myocardial viability as detected by positron emission tomography in patients with ischemic cardiomyopathy. Circulation 1999;99(22):2921–6.

[30] Wei L, Kadoya M, Momose M, et al. Serial assessment of left ventricular function in various patient groups with Tl-201 gated myocardial perfusion SPECT. Radiat Med 2007;25(2):65–72.

[31] Bell SP, Fabian J, Watkins MW, et al. Decrease in forces responsible for diastolic suction during

acute coronary occlusion. Circulation 1997;96(7): 2348–52.

[32] Firstenberg MS, Smedira NG, Greenberg NL, et al. Relationship between early diastolic intraventricular pressure gradients, an index of elastic recoil, and improvements in systolic and diastolic function. Circulation 2001;104(12 Suppl 1):I330–5.

[33] Uren NG, Melin JA, De Bruyne B, et al. Relation between myocardial blood flow and the severity of coronary-artery stenosis. N Engl J Med 1994; 330(25):1782–8.

[34] Di Carli M, Czernin J, Hoh CK, et al. Relation among stenosis severity, myocardial blood flow, and flow reserve in patients with coronary artery disease. Circulation 1995;91(7):1944–51.

[35] Cowie MR, Wood DA, Coats AJ, et al. Incidence and aetiology of heart failure; a population-based study. Eur Heart J 1999;20(6):421–8.

[36] Gheorghiade M, Bonow RO. Chronic heart failure in the United States: a manifestation of coronary artery disease. Circulation 1998;97(3):282–9.

[37] Levy D, Larson MG, Vasan RS, et al. The progression from hypertension to congestive heart failure. JAMA 1996;275(20):1557–62.

[38] Uretsky BF, Thygesen K, Armstrong PW, et al. Acute coronary findings at autopsy in heart failure patients with sudden death: results from the assessment of treatment with lisinopril and survival (ATLAS) trial. Circulation 2000;102(6):611–6.

[39] Repetto A, Dal Bello B, Pasotti M, et al. Coronary atherosclerosis in end-stage idiopathic dilated cardiomyopathy: an innocent bystander? Eur Heart J 2005;26(15):1519–27.

[40] Felker GM, Thompson RE, Hare JM, et al. Underlying causes and long-term survival in patients with initially unexplained cardiomyopathy. N Engl J Med 2000;342(15):1077–84.

[41] Hedrich O, Jacob M, Hauptman PJ. Progression of coronary artery disease in non-ischemic dilated cardiomyopathy. Coron Artery Dis 2004;15(5): 291–7.

[42] Graf S, Khorsand A, Gwechenberger M, et al. Typical chest pain and normal coronary angiogram: cardiac risk factor analysis versus PET for detection of microvascular disease. J Nucl Med 2007;48(2): 175–81.

[43] Qian JY, Ge JB, Fan B, et al. Identification of syndrome X using intravascular ultrasound imaging and Doppler flow mapping. Chin Med J (Engl) 2004;117(4):521–7.

[44] Bart BA, Shaw LK, McCants CB Jr, et al. Clinical determinants of mortality in patients with angiographically diagnosed ischemic or nonischemic cardiomyopathy. J Am Coll Cardiol 1997;30(4): 1002–8.

[45] Felker GM, Shaw LK, O'Connor CM. A standardized definition of ischemic cardiomyopathy for use in clinical research. J Am Coll Cardiol 2002;39(2): 210–8.

[46] Purek L, Laule-Kilian K, Christ A, et al. Coronary artery disease and outcome in acute congestive heart failure. Heart 2006;92(5):598–602.

[47] Yusuf S, Zhao F, Mehta SR, et al. Effects of clopidogrel in addition to aspirin in patients with acute coronary syndromes without ST-segment elevation. N Engl J Med 2001;345(7):494–502.

[48] Pfeffer MA, Braunwald E, Moye LA, et al. Effect of captopril on mortality and morbidity in patients with left ventricular dysfunction after myocardial infarction. Results of the survival and ventricular enlargement trial. The SAVE Investigators. N Engl J Med 1992;327(10):669–77.

[49] Yusuf S, Pepine CJ, Garces C, et al. Effect of enalapril on myocardial infarction and unstable angina in patients with low ejection fractions. Lancet 1992; 340(8829):1173–8.

[50] Pitt B, White H, Nicolau J, et al. Eplerenone reduces mortality 30 days after randomization following acute myocardial infarction in patients with left ventricular systolic dysfunction and heart failure. J Am Coll Cardiol 2005;46(3):425–31.

[51] Janosi A, Ghali JK, Herlitz J, et al. Metoprolol CR/XL in postmyocardial infarction patients with chronic heart failure: experiences from MERIT-HF. Am Heart J 2003;146(4):721–8.

[52] Effect of ramipril on mortality and morbidity of survivors of acute myocardial infarction with clinical evidence of heart failure. The Acute Infarction Ramipril Efficacy (AIRE) Study Investigators. Lancet 1993;342(8875):821–8.

[53] O'Connor CM, Velazquez EJ, Gardner LH, et al. Comparison of coronary artery bypass grafting versus medical therapy on long-term outcome in patients with ischemic cardiomyopathy (a 25-year experience from the Duke Cardiovascular Disease Databank). Am J Cardiol 2002;90(2): 101–7.

[54] Alderman EL, Fisher LD, Litwin P, et al. Results of coronary artery surgery in patients with poor left ventricular function (CASS). Circulation 1983; 68(4):785–95.

[55] Baker DW, Jones R, Hodges J, et al. Management of heart failure. III. The role of revascularization in the treatment of patients with moderate or severe left ventricular systolic dysfunction. JAMA 1994; 272(19):1528–34.

[56] Pigott JD, Kouchoukos NT, Oberman A, et al. Late results of surgical and medical therapy for patients with coronary artery disease and depressed left ventricular function. J Am Coll Cardiol 1985;5(5): 1036–45.

[57] Elefteriades JA, Tolis G Jr, Levi E, et al. Coronary artery bypass grafting in severe left ventricular dysfunction: excellent survival with improved ejection fraction and functional state. J Am Coll Cardiol 1993;22(5):1411–7.

[58] Kannel WB, Gordon T, Offutt D. Left ventricular hypertrophy by electrocardiogram. Prevalence,

[59] incidence, and mortality in the Framingham study. Ann Intern Med 1969;71(1):89–105.

[59] Kannel WB, Dannenberg AL, Levy D. Population implications of electrocardiographic left ventricular hypertrophy. Am J Cardiol 1987;60(17):85I–93I.

[60] Levy D, Anderson KM, Savage DD, et al. Echocardiographically detected left ventricular hypertrophy: prevalence and risk factors. The Framingham Heart Study. Ann Intern Med 1988;108(1):7–13.

[61] Urbina EM, Gidding SS, Bao W, et al. Effect of body size, ponderosity, and blood pressure on left ventricular growth in children and young adults in the Bogalusa Heart Study. Circulation 1995;91(9): 2400–6.

[62] Inouye I, Massie B, Loge D, et al. Abnormal left ventricular filling: an early finding in mild to moderate systemic hypertension. Am J Cardiol 1984;53(1): 120–6.

[63] Smith VE, Schulman P, Karimeddini MK, et al. Rapid ventricular filling in left ventricular hypertrophy: II. Pathologic hypertrophy. J Am Coll Cardiol 1985;5(4):869–74.

[64] Pearson AC, Gudipati C, Nagelhout D, et al. Echocardiographic evaluation of cardiac structure and function in elderly subjects with isolated systolic hypertension. J Am Coll Cardiol 1991;17(2):422–30.

[65] Devereux RB. Left ventricular diastolic dysfunction: early diastolic relaxation and late diastolic compliance. J Am Coll Cardiol 1989;13(2):337–9.

[66] Brucks S, Little WC, Chao T, et al. Contribution of left ventricular diastolic dysfunction to heart failure regardless of ejection fraction. Am J Cardiol 2005; 95(5):603–6.

[67] Marcus ML, Harrison DG, Chilian WM, et al. Alterations in the coronary circulation in hypertrophied ventricles. Circulation 1987;75(1 Pt 2):I19–25.

[68] Gandhi SK, Powers JC, Nomeir AM, et al. The pathogenesis of acute pulmonary edema associated with hypertension. N Engl J Med 2001;344(1):17–22.

[69] Gheorghiade M, Zannad F, Sopko G, et al. Acute heart failure syndromes: current state and framework for future research. Circulation 2005;112(25): 3958–68.

[70] Vasan RS, Larson MG, Leip EP, et al. Impact of high-normal blood pressure on the risk of cardiovascular disease. N Engl J Med 2001;345(18): 1291–7.

[71] Chobanian AV, Bakris GL, Black HR, et al. Seventh report of the Joint National Committee on Prevention, Detection, Evaluation, and Treatment of High Blood Pressure. Hypertension 2003;42(6):1206–52.

[72] Flegal KM, Carroll MD, Ogden CL, et al. Prevalence and trends in obesity among US adults, 1999–2000. JAMA 2002;288(14):1723–7.

[73] Kostis JB, Davis BR, Cutler J, et al. Prevention of heart failure by antihypertensive drug treatment in older persons with isolated systolic hypertension. SHEP Cooperative Research Group. JAMA 1997; 278(3):212–6.

[74] Dahlof B, Lindholm LH, Hansson L, et al. Morbidity and mortality in the Swedish Trial in Old Patients with Hypertension (STOP-Hypertension). Lancet 1991;338(8778):1281–5.

[75] Moser M, Hebert PR. Prevention of disease progression, left ventricular hypertrophy and congestive heart failure in hypertension treatment trials. J Am Coll Cardiol 1996;27(5):1214–8.

[76] Vasan RS, Levy D. The role of hypertension in the pathogenesis of heart failure. A clinical mechanistic overview. Arch Intern Med 1996;156(16): 1789–96.

[77] Yusuf S, Sleight P, Pogue J, et al. Effects of an angiotensin-converting-enzyme inhibitor, ramipril, on cardiovascular events in high-risk patients. The Heart Outcomes Prevention Evaluation Study Investigators. N Engl J Med 2000;342(3):145–53.

[78] Effect of enalapril on mortality and the development of heart failure in asymptomatic patients with reduced left ventricular ejection fractions. The SOLVD Investigators. N Engl J Med 1992;327(10): 685–91.

[79] Mathew J, Sleight P, Lonn E, et al. Reduction of cardiovascular risk by regression of electrocardiographic markers of left ventricular hypertrophy by the angiotensin-converting enzyme inhibitor ramipril. Circulation 2001;104(14):1615–21.

[80] Ingelsson E, Bjorklund-Bodegard K, Lind L, et al. Diurnal blood pressure pattern and risk of congestive heart failure. JAMA 2006;295(24): 2859–66.

[81] Vasan RS, Beiser A, Seshadri S, et al. Residual lifetime risk for developing hypertension in middle-aged women and men: The Framingham Heart Study. JAMA 2002;287(8):1003–10.

[82] Staessen JA, Gasowski J, Wang JG, et al. Risks of untreated and treated isolated systolic hypertension in the elderly: meta-analysis of outcome trials. Lancet 2000;355(9207):865–72.

[83] Stamler J, Stamler R, Neaton JD. Blood pressure, systolic and diastolic, and cardiovascular risks. US population data. Arch Intern Med 1993;153(5): 598–615.

[84] Brush JE Jr, Cannon RO III, Schenke WH, et al. Angina due to coronary microvascular disease in hypertensive patients without left ventricular hypertrophy. N Engl J Med 1988;319(20):1302–7.

[85] Bache RJ, Arentzen CE, Simon AB, et al. Abnormalities in myocardial perfusion during tachycardia in dogs with left ventricular hypertrophy: metabolic evidence for myocardial ischemia. Circulation 1984; 69(2):409–17.

[86] Zhang J, Merkle H, Hendrich K, et al. Bioenergetic abnormalities associated with severe left ventricular hypertrophy. J Clin Invest 1993;92(2):993–1003.

[87] Falk E, Shah PK, Fuster V. Coronary plaque disruption. Circulation 1995;92(3):657–71.

[88] Giannattasio C, Mangoni AA, Failla M, et al. Impaired radial artery compliance in normotensive subjects with familial hypercholesterolemia. Atherosclerosis 1996;124(2):249–60.

[89] van der Linde NA, Sijbrands EJ, Boomsma F, et al. Effect of low-density lipoprotein cholesterol on angiotensin II sensitivity: a randomized trial with fluvastatin. Hypertension 2006;47(6):1125–30.

[90] Leibovitz E, Beniashvili M, Zimlichman R, et al. Treatment with amlodipine and atorvastatin have additive effect in improvement of arterial compliance in hypertensive hyperlipidemic patients. Am J Hypertens 2003;16(9 Pt 1):715–8.

[91] Egashira K, Hirooka Y, Kai H, et al. Reduction in serum cholesterol with pravastatin improves endothelium-dependent coronary vasomotion in patients with hypercholesterolemia. Circulation 1994;89(6): 2519–24.

[92] Vasan RS, Evans JC, Larson MG, et al. Serum aldosterone and the incidence of hypertension in nonhypertensive persons. N Engl J Med 2004;351(1): 33–41.

[93] Newton-Cheh C, Guo CY, Gona P, et al. Clinical and genetic correlates of aldosterone-to-renin ratio and relations to blood pressure in a community sample. Hypertension 2007;49(4):846–56.

[94] Kathiresan S, Larson MG, Benjamin EJ, et al. Clinical and genetic correlates of serum aldosterone in the community: the Framingham Heart Study. Am J Hypertens 2005;18(5 Pt 1):657–65.

[95] Kathiresan S, Gona P, Larson MG, et al. Cross-sectional relations of multiple biomarkers from distinct biological pathways to brachial artery endothelial function. Circulation 2006;113(7):938–45.

[96] Wang TJ, Gona P, Larson MG, et al. Multiple biomarkers for the prediction of first major cardiovascular events and death. N Engl J Med 2006; 355(25):2631–9.

[97] Yusuf S, Reddy S, Ounpuu S, et al. Global burden of cardiovascular diseases: part I: general considerations, the epidemiologic transition, risk factors, and impact of urbanization. Circulation 2001; 104(22):2746–53.

[98] Kannel WB. Lessons from curbing the coronary artery disease epidemic for confronting the impending epidemic of heart failure. Med Clin North Am 2004;88(5):1129–33, ix.

ELSEVIER
SAUNDERS

CARDIOLOGY
CLINICS

Cardiol Clin 25 (2007) 497–506

Guidelines for the Management of Heart Failure: Differences in Guideline Perspectives

Mariell Jessup, MD*, Susan C. Brozena, MD

Hospital of the University of Pennsylvania, Philadelphia, PA, USA

In 1980, the American College of Cardiology (ACC) and the American Heart Association (AHA) formed a joint effort to develop practice guidelines for cardiovascular disease management. The rationale for this approach appears in the opening paragraphs of each ACC/AHA guideline published: "It is important that the medical profession play a significant role in critically evaluating the use of diagnostic procedures and therapies as they are introduced and tested in the detection, management, or prevention of disease states. Rigorous and expert analysis of the available data documenting relative benefits and risks of those procedures and therapies can produce helpful guidelines that improve the effectiveness of care, optimize patient outcomes, and favorably affect the overall cost of care by focusing resources on the most effective strategies" [1]. In short, the development of clinical or practice guidelines is thought to be a successful strategy for improving quality of care. Accordingly, many professional organizations, societies, institutions of health care or policy, and even countries have published practice guidelines on a variety of topics, including heart failure [2–6]. Table 1 lists a few recently published heart failure guidelines addressing chronic and acute heart failure. This list is far from complete and does not include the many guidelines written in languages other than English. Indeed, a quick search on the National Guideline Clearinghouse

Web site (www.guideline.gov) revealed 431 heart failure–related guidelines.

Essential guideline components

Sackett [7] defined guidelines as user-friendly statements that bring together the best external evidence and other knowledge necessary for decision making about a specific health problem. Sackett further suggested that good clinical guidelines have three essential properties: (1) guidelines ideally should define practice questions and explicitly identify all the decision options and outcomes; (2) guidelines should assess and summarize in an easily accessible format the best evidence about prevention, diagnosis, prognosis, therapy, harm, and cost-effectiveness; and (3) guidelines should identify the decision points at which the cited valid evidence needs to be integrated with individual clinical experience in deciding on a course of action. Using these criteria, practice guidelines optimally do not specify decisions one should make but rather outline the range of potential decisions to incorporate with clinical judgment and the patient's wishes and expectations [8]. Understandably, individual guideline writing groups might take exception to the dictates of these three critical properties. For example, professional societies may not want to tackle the difficult issues of cost-effectiveness, especially with respect to a class of drugs with many options on the market, such as the angiotensin-converting enzyme (ACE) inhibitors or angiotensin receptor blockers (ARBs). Are the less expensive, generic drugs as good as the more expensive brand name items? Conversely, governmental health and insurance guidelines may, by necessity, have to specifically address the thorny cost-effectiveness data or lack

* Corresponding author. Heart Failure/Transplant Program, 3400 Spruce Street, 6 Penn Tower, Philadelphia, PA 19104.

E-mail address: jessupm@uphs.upenn.edu (M. Jessup).

0733-8651/07/$ - see front matter © 2007 Elsevier Inc. All rights reserved.
doi:10.1016/j.ccl.2007.08.004

Table 1
Available international guidelines for management of heart failure

Sponsor	Citation
Chronic heart failure	
Scottish Intercollegiate Guidelines Network	Management of chronic heart failure: a national clinical guideline. Available at: www.sign.ac.uk. Accessed February 2007
Canadian Cardiovascular Society	Arnold JM, Liu P, Demers, et al. Canadian Cardiovascular Society Consensus Conference recommendations on heart failure 2006: diagnosis and management. Can J Cardiol 2006;22:23–45
Heart Failure Society of America	Adams KF, Lindenfeld J, Arnold JM, et al. Executive Summary: HFSA 2006. Comprehensive heart failure practice guidelines. J Cardiac Failure 2006;12:10–38
European Society of Cardiology	Swedberg K, Cleland J, Dargier H, et al. Guidelines for the diagnosis and treatment of chronic heart failure: executive summary (update 2005). Task Force on Chronic Heart Failure of the European Society of Cardiology. Eur Heart J 2005;26:1115–40
American College of Cardiology/American Heart Association	Hunt SA, Abraham WT, Chin MH, et al. ACC/AHA 2005 Guideline Update for the diagnosis and management of chronic heart failure in the adult. ACC/AHA Task Force on Practice Guidelines. Circulation 2005;112(12):E154–235
Royal College of Physicians	The National Collaborating Center for Chronic Conditions. Chronic Heart Failure: national clinical guideline for diagnosis and management in primary and secondary care. Royal College of Physicians 2003. Available at: www.rcplondon.ac.uk
Acute heart failure	
Canadian Cardiovascular Society	Arnold JM, Howlett JG, Dorian P, et al. Canadian Cardiovascular Society Consensus Conference recommendations on heart failure update 2007: prevention, management during intercurrent illness or acute decompensation, and use of biomarkers. Can J Cardiol 2007;23(1):21–45
European Society of Cardiology	Nieminen MS, Bohm M, Cowie MR, et al, The ESC Committee for Practice Guideline. Executive summary of the guidelines on the diagnosis and treatment of acute heart failure: the Task Force on Acute Heart Failure of the European Society of Cardiology. Eur Heart J 2005;26:384–416
Heart Failure Society of America	Adams KF, Lindenfeld J, Arnold JMO, et al. Executive Summary: HFSA 2006. Comprehensive heart failure practice guidelines. J Cardiac Failure 2006;12:10–38

thereof. The reason for the organization's need to elaborate a set of guidelines will, in part, determine how well the document adheres to the criteria outlined previously.

Similarities and differences in heart failure guidelines

The recent proliferation of heart failure guidelines has prompted an inevitable comparison between the recommendations found in one set with that in another [9]. Tables 2 and 3 depict comparisons for some of the more recent guideline publications for heart failure with systolic dysfunction and for heart failure with preserved left ventricular function, respectively. Fortunately, some fundamental commonalities exist among the guidelines for low ejection fraction heart failure. These commonalities include a mandated trial of ACE inhibitors and beta-blockers for all patients; however, even this consensus is lessened somewhat by the details discussed in the individual guidelines with respect to issues such as which beta-blockers should be used or the symptomatic status of the patient with systolic dysfunction (see Table 2). Examining the differences between guidelines for other forms of therapy or devices reveals many inconsistencies, not the least of which is the fact that some guidelines fail to address certain topics for lack of data, whereas others apply "expert opinion" to formulate a recommendation. Many writing groups use a specific vocabulary to express the level of evidence for a certain recommendation (eg, "should" or "might be effective") in addition to assigning a grade.

What are the reasons for the lack of uniformity between heart failure guidelines? Presumably, everyone has access to the same clinical trial publications. In a thoughtful editorial by McMurray and Swedberg [9], both of whom are prominent heart failure clinicians and trialists, several potential difficulties that face guideline writing committees were discussed. One major source of interpretive discrepancies is the increasing use of composite endpoints in heart failure trials. A new therapy, "Drug X," may reach a statistically significant outcome in a multicenter trial but only on the basis of a decrease in heart failure hospitalizations while no apparent effect on mortality is noted. Each guideline committee must then decide how to incorporate Drug X into their patient care recommendations. One approach might be to delineate how Drug X should be used to decrease heart failure hospitalizations. Another writing group might give Drug X a less strong mandate by the language used, such as "could consider" without mentioning the details of the trial's composite endpoint. A third committee might not mention Drug X at all until a definitive mortality trial was completed for the drug.

Another source for the lack of uniformity between guidelines is the increasing complexity of a heart failure regimen upon which new therapies must be added. For example, several important trials have examined the morbidity and mortality effect of an additional investigational treatment onto a baseline regimen of diuretics, beta-blockers, and ACE inhibitors in symptomatic patients. These trials have explored interventions with ARBs, aldosterone antagonists, implantable defibrillators (ICDs), cardiac resynchronization, and a specially formulated hydralazine-nitrate combination. Nevertheless, no trials have addressed which of these successful interventions should be tried first for an individual patient who continues to be symptomatic despite optimal therapy. Guideline

committees must then struggle to make reasonable interpretations of the data as they organize their report. Some committees will scrutinize the study population of each trial and use the specific differences found to develop recommendations. Other writing groups will shrink from any prioritization of next-step therapy because of inadequate evidence.

Certain drugs and devices were tested many years ago in heart failure patients managed on diuretics alone or on ACE inhibitors but not beta-blockers. Are the outcomes of these trials valid for the current population of patients who may be on several additional drugs? Writing committees may consider these historical comparisons with widely divergent opinions. Yet another area in which guideline writing committees disagree is their willingness to apply therapies to all heart failure patients if they have only been studied in a specific subset of patients. Some examples of such dilemmas include the use of ICDs in patients who have never had heart failure symptoms, the use of spironolactone in asymptomatic patients, and the use of hydralazine-nitrates in patients other than African Americans. Achieving a consensus on these difficult items and scores of other equally contentious topics is unlikely.

Implementation of the guidelines

Even if all of the heart failure guidelines were identical (which would make the redundancy of guidelines an important issue), the wisdom contained in each document must be disseminated to, and embraced by, the practicing clinician. Predictably, there is an extensive body of literature addressing the most efficacious methods to implement guideline recommendations, some of which is summarized in the ACC/AHA heart failure document [1]. Basic physician education and passive dissemination of guidelines alone are generally insufficient to sustain quality improvement; rather, the distribution of the guideline information must be accompanied by more intensive educational and behavioral interventions to maximize the chances of improving physician practice patterns.

A commonly cited barrier to the implementation of guideline recommendations is the perception that the typical patient with heart failure is dissimilar to the patient enrolled in the heart failure trials upon which the evidence-based recommendations are derived [10,11]. Indeed, it is true that many of the large multicenter heart failure trials

Table 2
Comparison of recommendations from international guidelines for treatment of chronic heart failure due to left ventricular systolic dysfunction

Topic discussed	Scottish Intercollegiate Guidelines Network 2007	Canadian Cardiovascular Society 2006	Heart Failure Society of America 2006	European Society of Cardiology 2005	American College of Cardiology/American Heart Association 2005
ACE inhibitors	For all with or without symptoms	For all with LVEF ≤40%	For all with or without symptoms with LVEF ≤40%	First-line drug (IA) when LVEF <40%–45% with or without symptoms; Target doses given	Stage A appropriate; Stage B,C,D indicated
Beta-blockers	For all as soon as condition is stable; Recommend bisoprolol, carvedilol, or nebivolol	For all with LVEF ≤40%	Routine treatment in all patients with LVSD; In combination with ACE inhibitor, all patients post MI with LVEF ≤40%; No specific drugs mentioned	For all NYHA class II–IV with reduced LVEF; All patients with or without symptomatic heart failure following acute MI; Recommend bisoprolol, carvedilol, metoprolol succinate, or nebivolol	Stage B, all patients post MI; Stage B,C,D, all patients; Use one of three approved in United States: bisoprolol, carvedilol, or sustained-release metoprolol
ARBs	If intolerant to ACE inhibitor; May add candesartan to ACE inhibitor and beta-blocker only in consultation with a specialist	If intolerant to ACE inhibitor; May be adjunctive to ACE inhibitor if patient cannot tolerate beta-blockers	If intolerant to ACE inhibitor	Alternative if intolerant to ACE inhibitor	Stage A can be useful; Stage B,C,D if intolerant of ACE inhibitor
Digoxin	Add-on therapy in NSR, if still symptomatic after optimal therapy	Patients with NSR with continued moderate-to-severe symptoms despite optimized medical therapy to relieve symptoms and reduce hospitalizations; Chronic AF and poor rate control; Trough level can be <1 ng/mL to achieve optimal benefit with reduced risk of side effects	Consider for patients with LVEF ≤40% with symptomatic HF; Daily dose should be 0.125 mg daily; Recommend serum trough level <1.0 ng/mL	Indicated with AF and may reduce hospitalizations and worsening HF, hospitalizations in patients with LVSD and NSR, and with severe HF; Daily dose up to 0.25 mg, lower in the elderly; No target trough level noted	Stage C, can be beneficial to decrease hospitalizations

Diuretics	For all with dyspnea or edema	Loop diuretic for most with symptoms of congestion Others may be added PRN to augment diuresis	Loop diuretics when symptoms due to sodium and water retention Others may be added PRN to augment	Essential for symptomatic treatment when fluid overload is present	For patients with fluid retention
Aldosterone antagonists	Spironolactone following specialist advice if moderate-to-severe symptoms Eplerenone post MI if LVEF ≤40% and diabetes or clinical signs of HF	Spironolactone for patients with LVEF <30% and severe symptoms despite optimized treatment Also in patients with LVEF <30% and HF post MI if serum creatinine acceptable	NYHA class III–IV, LVEF ≤35% while receiving standard therapy	Recommended in addition to ACE inhibitor and beta-blocker and diuretics in advanced HF with systolic dysfunction and after MI with LV dysfunction, HF symptoms, or diabetes	Stage C,D, for moderate-to-severe symptoms in those who can be carefully monitored
Hydralazine/ isosorbide dinitrate	If intolerant of or symptomatic despite ACE inhibitor or ARB, and for African Americans with symptomatic HF	If intolerant of or symptomatic despite ACE inhibitor or ARB, and for African Americans with symptomatic HF	If intolerant of or symptomatic despite ACE inhibitor or ARB, and for African Americans with symptomatic HF	If intolerant to ACE inhibitor or ARBs	Stage C, if symptomatic despite ACE inhibitor and beta-blocker, if intolerant of ACE inhibitor or ARB, and for African Americans with symptomatic HF
Nitrates	For angina	To relieve orthopnea, PND, angina, exercise-induced dyspnea Not recommended for use as primary therapy		For concomitant angina or relief of dyspnea	
Calcium antagonists	Avoid except for amlodipine if angina present			Not recommended Amlodipine or felodipine are safe alternatives if angina or hypertension persist	Stage B,C,D, not indicated

(continued on next page)

Table 2 (*continued*)

Topic discussed	Scottish Intercollegiate Guidelines Network 2007	Canadian Cardiovascular Society 2006	Heart Failure Society of America 2006	European Society of Cardiology 2005	American College of Cardiology/American Heart Association 2005
Warfarin		All patients with HF and AF Not routinely recommended for patients in NSR, but should be considered in those with documented intracardiac thrombus, spontaneous echo contrast, or severe reduction in LV systolic function when thrombus cannot be excluded	All with HF and AF, history of emboli, CVA, TIA For 3 months post large anterior MI or recent MI with documented thrombus Presence of LV thrombus and LVSD May also be considered in DCM and LVEF ≤35%	Indicated if AF, previous thromboembolic event, mobile LV thrombus	If patient has AF or previous thromboembolic event
Antiplatelet therapy	No firm evidence to support the use or withdrawal of aspirin in patients with HF	Aspirin if clear indication for secondary prevention of atherosclerotic disease	Patients with HF and ischemic CMP Not recommended for those patients with IDCM Use with ACE inhibitor if indication for both exist Use low dose	Avoid aspirin in patients with worsening or repeated episodes HF	Antiplatelet agents should be prescribed in those patients with underlying coronary disease
Antiarrhythmics			Not for primary prevention sudden death Amiodarone may be used in patients with repetitive ICD discharges	Avoid class I amiodarone to treat atrial or ventricular arrhythmias Beta-blockers reduce sudden death in HF	Avoid IA, IC Amiodarone has neutral effects on survival in patients with HF and LVSD
Oxygen	No evidence of benefit for HF		Not recommended	No application in chronic HF	
Inotropes		Should be reserved for patients with acute HF and signs of low or very low cardiac output	For acute decompensated with diminished peripheral perfusion	Recommend against oral inotropes	Long-term use of an infusion for palliation only

Non-cardiac drugs to avoid	St. John's wort due to drug interactions, tricyclic antidepressants	Thiazolidinediones, antiarrhythmics, doxorubicin, NSAIDs, celecoxib, penicillins, corticosteroids, tricyclic antidepressants, zidovudine, licorice, venlafaxine	Not addressed	NSAIDs, COX inhibitors, tricyclic antidepressants, corticosteroids, lithium	Hormonal therapies (growth or thyroid), nutritional supplements, thiazolidinediones if moderate-to-severe symptoms
Use of alcohol	Refrain from excessive use; abstain if alcohol-related heart disease	Not addressed	Discouraged in all patients; abstinence if previous excessive use	One beer or 1–2 glasses wine daily unless alcohol-related CMP	Refrain from excessive use; abstain if alcohol-related heart disease
Nonpharmacologic[a]	Addressed	Addressed	Addressed	Addressed	Addressed
Cardiac resynchronization	NSR, drug-refractory symptoms, class III–IV, LVEF ≤35%, QRS duration ≥120msec	NYHA III–IV despite optimized medical therapy, in NSR, QRS duration ≥120 msec and LVEF ≤35%	LVEF ≤35%, with LV dilatation > 5.5 cm, QRS duration ≥120 msec, class III symptoms Not recommended if asymptomatic or class II	Low LVEF, class III–IV symptoms, QRS duration ≥120 msec	Stage C, LVEF ≤35%, class III–IV symptoms, QRS duration ≥120 msec
Primary prevention ICD	Not addressed	Patients with ischemic heart disease, mild-to-moderate HF symptoms, LVEF ≤30%, at least 1 mo after MI or 3 mo after revascularization Patients with non-ischemic CMP, NYHA class II–III, LVEF ≤ 30%, or LVEF 31%–35%	Patients with LVEF ≤30% and may be considered if LVEF 31%–35% with mild-to-moderate symptoms Not recommended in severe HF if no chance of improvement	Selected patients with LVEF <30% to 35%, on optimal medical therapy, and >40 d post MI	Stage B, 40 d post MI and LVEF ≤ 30% Stage C, LVEF ≤30%, class II–III symptoms on optimal therapy
HF in the elderly	Addressed	Addressed	Addressed	Addressed	Addressed
End-of-life care	Addressed	Addressed	Addressed	Not addressed	Addressed

Abbreviations: AF, atrial fibrillation; CMP, cardiomyopathy; CVA, cerebrovascular accident; DCM, dilated cardiomyopathy; HF, heart failure; ICD, implantable cardioverter defibrillator; IDCM, idiopathic dilated cardiomyopathy; LVSD, left systolic dysfunction; LVEF, left ventricular ejection fraction; MI, myocardial infarction; NSR, normal sinus rhythm; NYHA, New York Heart Association; PND, paroxysmal nocturnal dyspnea; TIA, transient ischemic attack.

[a] Education, weight monitoring, sodium and fluid restriction, smoking cessation, exercise.

Table 3
Comparison of recommendations from international guidelines for treatment of chronic heart failure with preserved left ventricular ejection fraction

Topic discussed	Scottish Intercollegiate Guidelines Network 2007	Canadian Cardiovascular Society 2006	Heart Failure Society of America 2006	European Society of Cardiology 2005	American College of Cardiology/ American Heart Association 2005
ACE inhibitors	No good evidence	For most patients	All patients with other risk factors such as atherosclerotic disease or diabetes	May improve relaxation	Might be effective to control HF
Beta-blockers	No good evidence	For most patients	For symptomatic patients who have prior MI, hypertension, or atrial fibrillation	Use to lower heart rate and increase diastolic filling time	Might be effective to control HF
ARBs	No good evidence	Consider to reduce HF hospitalization	All patients with LVDD	High dose may decrease hospitalizations	Might be effective to control HF
Digoxin		May be considered to minimize symptoms			Use is not well established
Diuretics	No good evidence	Use to control pulmonary congestion and edema	Necessary with fluid overload, but use cautiously to avoid lowering preload	Necessary with fluid overload, but use cautiously to avoid lowering preload	Necessary with fluid overload, but use cautiously to avoid lowering preload
Calcium antagonists	No good evidence	May be considered to minimize symptoms	For control of rate in atrial fibrillation, angina, hypertension	Verapamil-type drugs may be used	Might be effective to minimize symptoms

Abbreviations: HF, heart failure; LVDD, left ventricular diastolic dysfunction; MI, myocardial infarction.

performed over the past 2 decades failed to enroll a large percentage of women, ethnic or racial minorities, the very elderly, or patients with important comorbidities such as renal insufficiency. Perhaps the most important exclusion has been the patient with heart failure and preserved systolic function, a group that accounts for almost 50% of all heart failure hospitalizations [12,13]. Efforts are now being made to examine the therapeutic efficacy of some heart failure treatments in these important subpopulations [14]. Several additional factors may explain the reported underuse of evidence-based treatment, such as lack of knowledge, lack of expertise in the use of such drugs, lack of time, and economic restraints.

Whatever the reasons for the underuse of highly effective treatments, it is imperative that we begin to understand and address the root causes [15]. A recent study highlights the difficulties in assessing cause and effect. In a subgroup of the Euro Heart Failure Survey patients, a number of persons were identified to be similar to patients enrolled in the landmark ACE inhibitor and beta-blocker trials. Of these trial-eligible patients, hardly one half were prescribed a beta-blocker, and the doses of ACE inhibitors and beta-blockers used were lower than those proven to be effective in large controlled clinical trials. It was concluded that the lack of similarity between patients with heart failure in clinical practice and those in clinical trials does not adequately explain the underuse of therapy [16]. In a related study using additional data from the Euro Heart Failure survey, Lainscak and colleagues [17] noted that relevant comorbidity is responsible for a substantial reduction in the prescription of ACE inhibitors and beta-blockers. They noted in their discussion that international guidelines have been successful in creating a relatively uniform approach to the management of important aspects of treatment for heart failure across national borders; however, they cautioned that although co-morbidity indicates the need for greater caution, greater expert care, and more intensive monitoring of heart failure drugs, it is often not a valid reason for withholding lifesaving therapy.

Newer heart failure initiatives are achieving two goals: (1) surveying the use of lifesaving therapy and (2) promoting the uptake of these treatments. As an example, the Registry to Improve the Use of Evidence-Based Heart Failure Therapies in the Outpatient Setting (IMPROVE HF) is the first large-scale, comprehensive registry and process-of-care improvement initiative for ambulatory heart failure patients. It seeks to enhance quality of care and clinical outcomes by identifying the current management of outpatients with systolic heart failure and promoting the adoption of evidence-based, guideline-recommended therapies in the treatment of eligible outpatients. The program includes educational workshops, guideline-based treatment algorithms, and the provision of com-prehensive disease management tools. IMPROVE HF will also provide physicians and health care providers with performance feedback in bench-marked quality reports based on chart audits to help guide their practice [18]. This registry is one ef-fort to incorporate the many important lessons gleaned from randomized clinical trials into heart failure practice guidelines that are ultimately ap-plied to individual patients.

Heart failure practice guidelines evolve after tedious, expensive, and often mundane clinical trials are completed. Their completion involves the willing donation of many hours of typically uncompensated collaboration by heart failure ex-perts. Their dissemination requires additional hours of education and feedback, examining out-comes on a variety of endpoints. What remains to be done is the documentation that applying certain principles of practice will enhance patient quality and quantity of life [19,20].

References

[1] Hunt SA, Abraham WT, Chin MH, et al. ACC/ AHA 2005 Guideline Update for the Diagnosis and Management of Chronic Heart Failure in the Adult: a report of the American College of Cardiology/American Heart Association Task Force on Practice Guidelines (Writing Committee to Update the 2001 Guidelines for the Evaluation and Management of Heart Failure). Developed in collaboration with the American College of Chest Physicians and the International Society for Heart and Lung Transplantation: endorsed by the Heart Rhythm Society. Circulation 2005;112(12): E154–235.

[2] Adams KF, Lindenfeld J, Arnold JM, et al. Execu-tive Summary: HFSA 2006. Comprehensive heart failure practice guidelines. J Cardiac Failure 2006; 12:10–38.

[3] Arnold JM, Howlett JG, Dorian P, et al. Canadian Cardiovascular Society Consensus Conference rec-ommendations on heart failure update 2007: preven-tion, management during intercurrent illness or acute decompensation, and use of biomarkers. Can J Cardiol 2007;23(1):21–45.

[4] Arnold JM, Liu P, Demers C, et al. Canadian Car-diovascular Society Consensus Conference recom-mendations on heart failure 2006: diagnosis and management [erratum appears in Can J Cardiol 2006 Mar 1;22(3):271]. Can J Cardiol 2006;22(1): 23–45.

[5] Nieminen MS, Bohm M, Cowie MR, et al. Executive summary of the guidelines on the diagnosis and treatment of acute heart failure: the Task Force on Acute Heart Failure of the European Society of Car-diology. Eur Heart J 2005;26(4):384–416.

[6] Swedberg K, Cleland J, Dargie H, et al. Guidelines for the diagnosis and treatment of chronic heart fail-ure: executive summary (update 2005). The Task Force for the Diagnosis and Treatment of Chronic Heart Failure of the European Society of Cardiol-ogy. Eur Heart J 2005;26(11):1115–40.

[7] Sackett DL. Evidence-based medicine. Spine 1998; 23(10):1085–6.

[8] Ricci S, Celani MG, Righetti E. Development of clinical guidelines: methodological and practical is-sues. Neurol Sci 2006;27(Suppl 3):S228–30.

[9] McMurray J, Swedberg K. Treatment of chronic heart failure: a comparison between the major guide-lines. Eur Heart J 2006;27(15):1773–7.

[10] MacIntyre K, Capewell S, Stewart S, et al. Evidence of improving prognosis in heart failure: trends in case fatality in 66,547 patients hospitalized between 1986 and 1995. Circulation 2000;102(10):1126–31.

[11] Konstam M. Progress in heart failure management? Lessons from the real world. Circulation 2000;102: 1076–8.

[12] Owan T, Hodge D, Herges R, et al. Trends in prev-alence and outcome of heart failure with preserved ejection fraction. N Engl J Med 2006;355:251–9.

[13] Bhatia R, Tu J, Lee D, et al. Outcome of heart failure with preserved ejection fraction in a population-based study. N Engl J Med 2006;355:260–9.

[14] Manna DR, Bruijnzeels MA, Mokkink HG, et al. Ethnic specific recommendations in clinical practice

guidelines: a first exploratory comparison between guidelines from the USA, Canada, the UK, and the Netherlands [see comment]. Qual Saf Health Care 2003;12(5):353–8.

[15] Fonarow GC. How well are chronic heart failure patients being managed? Rev Cardiovasc Med 2006; 7(Suppl 1):S3–11.

[16] Lenzen MJ, Boersma E, Reimer WJ, et al. Under-utilization of evidence-based drug treatment in patients with heart failure is only partially explained by dissimilarity to patients enrolled in landmark trials: a report from the Euro Heart Survey on Heart Failure [see comment]. Eur Heart J 2005;26(24): 2706–13.

[17] Lainscak M, Cleland JG, Lenzen MJ, et al. International variations in the treatment and co-morbidity of left ventricular systolic dysfunction: data from the EuroHeart Failure Survey. Eur J Heart Fail 2007;9(3):292–9.

[18] Fonarow GC, Yancy CW, Albert NM, et al. Improving the use of evidence-based heart failure therapies in the outpatient setting: the IMPROVE HF performance improvement registry. Am Heart J 2007;154(1):12–38.

[19] Fonarow GC, Heywood JT, Heidenreich PA, et al. Investigators ASACa. Temporal trends in clinical characteristics, treatments, and outcomes for heart failure hospitalizations, 2002 to 2004: findings from Acute Decompensated Heart Failure National Registry (ADHERE). Am Heart J 2007;153(6):1021–8.

[20] Fonarow GC, Abraham WT, Albert NM, et al. Association between performance measures and clinical outcomes for patients hospitalized with heart failure. JAMA 2007;297(1):61–70.

Applying Hypertension Guidelines to Reduce the Burden of Heart Failure

Ragavendra R. Baliga, MD, MBA, FRCP, FACC

The Ohio State University, Columbus, OH, USA

Hypertension is the most common risk factor for heart failure, accounting for 39% of cases in men and 59% in women, and it contributes to a large proportion of heart failure cases [1]. High blood pressure confers a two- to threefold increase in risk for occurrence of heart failure [1]. Hypertension is also associated with development of heart failure in elderly persons and African Americans. Because approximately one fourth of the American population has hypertension and the lifetime risk of developing hypertension in the United States exceeds 75%, strategies to control blood pressure are an integral part of any effort to prevent heart failure [2]. The true incidence of heart failure has declined in women and has remained unchanged in men over the past 50 years (Fig. 1) [3]. According to the Joint National Committee (JNC7) within the last two decades, better treatment of hypertension has been associated with a considerable reduction in the hospital case fatality rate for heart failure (Fig. 2). The prevalence and hospitalization rates of heart failure, in which most patients have hypertension before developing heart failure, continue to increase, however (Fig. 3), because improved treatment has resulted in an increase in life expectancy [4].

Heart failure has been shown to be associated with systolic blood pressure, diastolic blood pressure, and pulse pressure [5]. Increases in systolic blood pressure and pulse pressure are associated linearly with the risk of heart failure without evidence of a threshold, whereas diastolic blood pressure and the risk of heart failure have a U-shaped association [6–8]. The added risk

conferred by increased pulse pressure is not solely due to isolated systolic elevation of blood pressure but a combination of an increase in systolic pressure and a fall in diastolic pressure—a reflection of increased hemodynamic load on the left ventricle.

Hypertensive heart disease includes increased left ventricular mass (Fig. 4), left ventricular diastolic dysfunction and left ventricular systolic dysfunction. Increased left ventricular mass is associated with a greater risk of heart failure, with the relative risk higher in younger individuals and the absolute risk higher in the older age group [9]. The risk of heart failure with left ventricular hypertrophy is independent of its association with hypertension. The relative risk of mortality increases twofold in patients with underlying coronary artery disease and fourfold in patients with normal coronary arteries [10,11]. In the Framingham study over a 4-year follow-up period, with each 50 g/m^2 increase in left ventricular mass there was a 1.57-fold increase in risk of cardiovascular disease for women and 1.49-fold increase in risk for men. The impact on cardiovascular morality was even more significant, with a 1.73-fold relative risk for men with each 50 g/m^2 and 2.12-fold risk for women [12].

Large community-based studies have shown that hypertension is a risk factor for heart failure in patients with and without systolic dysfunction [1,13]. Forty percent to 50% of patients who have heart failure have normal left ventricular ejection fraction. These patients typically have hypertension and left ventricular hypertrophy and are more likely to be women [14,15]. In the Olmsted County, Minnesota study of 216 patients evaluated, 52% had hypertension and 137 patients

---

E-mail address: ragavendra.baliga@osumc.edu

0733-8651/07/$ - see front matter © 2007 Elsevier Inc. All rights reserved.
doi:10.1016/j.ccl.2007.09.005

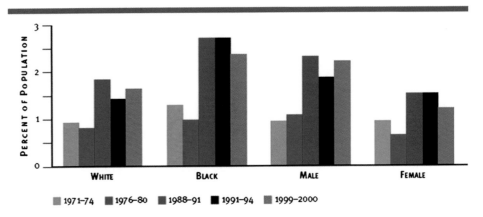

■ 1971–74   ■ 1976–80   ■ 1988–91   ■ 1991–94   ■ 1999–2000

Age-adjusted to 2000 U.S. census population.

Note: White and Black in 1999–2000 exclude Hispanics.

Fig. 1. Prevalence of congestive heart failure by race and gender, ages 25–74 years: United States, 1971–74 to 1999–2000. (*Adapted from* National Heart, Lung, and Blood Institute. Morbidity and mortality: 2002 chart book on cardiovascular, lung, and blood diseases. http://www.nhlbi.nih.gov/resources/docs/cht-book.htm, accessed November 2003; and M. Wolz and T. Thom, 1999–2000 unpublished data, National Heart, Lung, and Blood Institute, June 2003.)

underwent evaluation of left ventricular systolic function [13]. Hypertension was present in 58% of the patients with left ventricular systolic function more than 50% and in 53% of the patients with left ventricular systolic function less than 50%. In the Framingham study, after adjusting for risk factors for systolic heart failure, the risk of developing systolic heart failure in patients who had hypertension compared with patients who were normotensive was nearly twofold in men and threefold in women. Using multivariate analysis, these investigators reported that hypertension was the highest risk factor for systolic

heart failure, accounting for 59% of the cases in women and 39% of the cases in men [1]. The prognosis for patients with hypertension with newly diagnosed systolic heart failure was poor in the Framingham and Olmsted County studies—less than 35% 5-year survival rate.

Management

Among individuals who have hypertension, comorbidities such as diabetes, left ventricular hypertrophy, myocardial infarction, and valvular heart disease predict increased risk for heart

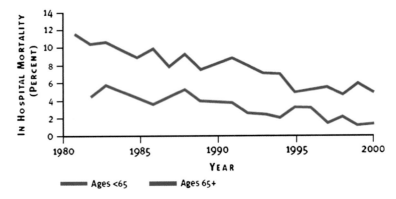

━━━ Ages <65   ━━━ Ages 65+

Fig. 2. Hospital case fatality rates for congestive heart failure for patients aged younger than 65 years and 65 years and older: United States, 1981–2000. (*Adapted from* National Heart, Lung, and Blood Institute. Morbidity and mortality: 2002 chart book on cardiovascular, lung, and blood diseases. http://www.nhlbi.nih.gov/resources/docs//cht-book.htm. Accessed November 2003.)

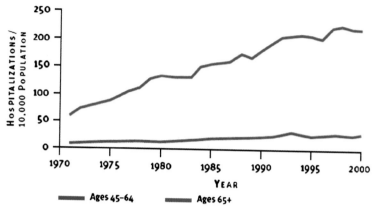

Fig. 3. Hospitalization rates for congestive heart failure in patients aged 45 to 64 years and 65 years and older: United States, 1971–2000. (*Adapted from* National Heart, Lung, and Blood Institute. Morbidity and mortality: 2002 chart book on cardiovascular, lung, and blood diseases. http://www.nhlbi.nih.gov/resources/docs//cht-book.htm. Accessed November 2003.)

failure. Survival after the onset of hypertensive heart failure may be dismal; only 24% of men and 31% of women survive 5 years. The relationship between blood pressure and risk of cardiovascular disease events is continuous, consistent, and independent of other risk factors—the higher the blood pressure, the greater the chance of heart failure. In the last 20 years, better management of elevated blood pressure has resulted in a considerable reduction in the hospital case fatality rate for heart failure. Keeping this in mind "The Seventh Report of the Joint National Committee on Prevention, Detection, Evaluation, and Treatment of High Blood Pressure: the JNC7 Report" [16] has opined that preventive strategies directed toward earlier and more aggressive blood pressure control are likely to offer the greatest promise for reducing the incidence of heart failure and consequent morbidity and mortality.

Systolic and diastolic heart failure, like other comorbidities associated with hypertension, is a consequence of systolic hypertension [1,17]. JNC7 focuses on the aggressive lowering of systolic and diastolic blood pressure and hyperlipidemia [18–20]. Further lowering of blood pressure is recommended in patients with accompanying cardiovascular risk factors, such as diabetes mellitus. Several studies have shown that optimal blood pressure control decreases the risk of new heart failure by approximately 50% [21]. The benefits of treating blood pressure in patients who have had a prior acute myocardial infarction are substantial, with an 81% reduction in the incidence of heart failure [20].

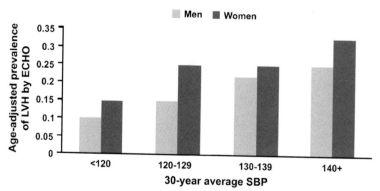

Fig. 4. Prevalence of left ventricular hypertrophy as a function of 30-year average systolic blood pressure. The Framingham Heart Study. (*From* Lauer MS, Anderson KM, Levy D. Influence of contemporary versus 30-year blood pressure levels on left ventricular mass and geometry: the Framingham Heart Study J Am Coll Cardiol 1991;18:1287–94; with permission.)

The management of hypertension involves achieving optimal blood pressure reduction through lifestyle changes and pharmacotherapy. The choice of therapy is determined by the presence of accompanying comorbidities, including coronary artery disease, renal disease, diabetes mellitus, and metabolic syndrome. (The latter includes any three of the following criteria: hypertension, central abdominal adiposity, low high-density lipoproteins, elevated triglycerides, and fasting hyperglycemia.) The JNC7 has recommended that target levels of blood pressure be lower in patients with associated major cardio-vascular risk factors, particularly in persons who have diabetes mellitus [22,23].

Lifestyle

In the JNC7 report, the term "prehypertension" was introduced to designate individuals whose systolic blood pressure levels are in the range of 120 to 139 mm Hg and diastolic blood pressure levels are between 80 and 89 mm Hg because (1) blood pressure usually increases with age, (2) more than 90% of the Framingham Heart Study cohort whose blood pressure was normal at age 55 ultimately developed hypertension in their lifetime, and (3) the risk of cardiovascular disease in adults between ages 40 and 80 increases progressively from levels as low as 115/75 mm Hg upward, with a doubling of the incidence of coronary artery disease and stroke for every 20/10 mm Hg increment of blood pressure. Using data from the 1999 to 2000 National Health and Nutrition Survey (NHANES), the prevalence of prehypertension is estimated to be 70 million individuals older than age 20. The JNC7 report recommends the adoption of healthy lifestyles in persons who have prehypertension to lower blood pressure, except in individuals who have accompanying diabetes or chronic renal disease in whom pharmacotherapy is also advocated. The epidemic of obesity suggests that adoption of a healthy lifestyle is the logical best step in these patients. A healthy lifestyle not only should lower blood pressure but also favorably impact diabetes, obesity, and dyslipidemia. It has been hypothesized that lowering salt intake should lower hypertension and accompanying left ventricular function in animal models.

Approximately 30% to 40% of patients with heart failure have normal left ventricular systolic function and has been to be shown to be due to diastolic dysfunction [24–27]. Morbidity and mortality in these patients are similar to that of patients who have heart failure with left ventricular systolic dysfunction [28,29]. Patients who have prehypertension and hypertension are at increased risk of developing diastolic dysfunction and left ventricular hypertrophy [30]. When blood pressure is untreated or poorly controlled, left ventricular hypertrophy is a major risk for dilated cardiomyopathy [12]. Approximately 11% to 15% of individuals with diastolic dysfunction develop heart failure over a 5-year follow-up period [31]. Progressive diastolic dysfunction is thought to be one of the key pathophysiologic mechanisms linking prehypertension and hypertension to diastolic heart failure. The ingestion of salt has been associated with elevated blood pressure, left ventricular hypertrophy, diastolic dysfunction, and heart failure [32–35]. Experimental evidence suggests a relationship between salt intake and an increase in myocardial mass and cardiac fibrosis. Restriction of salt has been shown to lower blood pressure [36–38]. Several studies have suggested a significant and independent association between dietary sodium intake and left ventricular hypertrophy [39–42]. Impaired left ventricular diastolic filling also has been shown to correlate with sodium excretion or blood pressure sodium sensitivity [35,43].

Several studies have reported the effectiveness of dietary approaches alone or in combination with other lifestyle modifications to reduce blood pressure in individuals who have prehypertension and hypertension [44]. JNC7 highlights the fact that weight loss of as little as 10 lb (4.5 kg) reduces blood pressure or prevents hypertension in a large proportion of the overweight individuals. It also stresses the importance of maintaining ideal body weight. When diet was modified in the Optimal Macro-Nutrient Intake Heart study to provide more protein and unsaturated fat and fewer carbohydrates, significant reductions in blood pressure were achieved. The PREMIER trial investigated the combined effects of diet, physical activity, and weight reduction in three groups of patients who had prehypertension and hypertension over an 18-month period [45,46]. In the group that received infrequent counseling sessions on modifying their lifestyles, the average decrease in blood pressure was 7.4/5.2 mm Hg. Patients who were provided with several group and individual counseling sessions showed an average reduction of 8.6/7.3 mm Hg. The third group, which differed from the second in that the subjects were also advised to adopt the

Dietary Approaches to Stop Hypertension (DASH) diet, showed an average blood pressure fall of 9.5/6.2 mm Hg. The DASH eating plan resulted in significant reduction in blood pressures independent of salt intake [47]. Although the DASH diet caused significant reductions in blood pressure across all population age groups independent of salt intake, the greatest effect on blood pressure was achieved by a combination of low salt intake and the DASH diet in the more recent DASH sodium study [38], whereas an increase in fruits and vegetables alone had no significant effect on blood pressure in individuals without hypertension in the original DASH study [48]. The totality of evidence for reducing salt is stronger than any other dietary constituents (eg, fruits and vegetables), but unlike reducing solely dietary salt, it requires major changes in eating habits. From a public health and clinical perspective, one of the most attainable strategies is to target salt hidden in processed foods, such as fast foods, TV dinners, and restaurant meals, which is approximately 80% of the excess salt consumed. If small reductions (10%–20%) were pursued, they would be detected by human taste receptors and should require minimal adaptation of food technology processes. If such reductions were repeated every 1 to 2 years, potentially the intake of salt could be reduced by approximately 6 g/d [49]. Reduction of salt should result in a substantial decrease in blood pressure in patients who have prehypertension, reduce the accompanying changes in left ventricular diastolic function, and prevent progression to heart failure. JNC7 recommends that dietary sodium be reduced to 100 mmol/d or less (2.4 g sodium).

Reduction of dietary salt in patients who have hypertension and are receiving antihypertensive medications provides additional benefits in terms of blood pressure control with diuretics, angiotensin-converting enzyme (ACE) inhibitors, and beta-blockers but not calcium-channel blockers. In one large study there was an additional 3 mm Hg decrease in diastolic blood pressure with reduced salt intake in patients on diuretic and beta-blocker therapy [50]. Another study showed that a low-salt diet provided an additional 4 mm Hg/2 mm Hg decrease in systolic blood and diastolic blood pressure, respectively, with beta-blocker and diuretic therapy [51]. A separate study showed that patients who had hypertension and were on diuretic therapy also benefited from salt reduction [52]. The blood pressure–lowering effects of salt reduction have been demonstrated

with patients who have hypertension who are on ACE inhibitor therapy. Two separate groups have shown that moderate salt reduction resulted in additional decreases in blood pressure in patients receiving captopril [53,54]. In a third study, when a low-salt diet was used with captopril treatment there was an additional reduction of 4 mm Hg/3 mm Hg in systolic and diastolic blood pressure, respectively [55]. The beneficial effect of dietary salt reduction on reducing blood pressure does not seem to affect patients who have hypertension who take calcium-channel blockers. The greatest reduction in blood pressure with calcium-channel blockers was seen in patients on a high-salt diet rather than a low-salt diet [56,57]. The additive effect of salt restriction leads to a further decrease of 3 to 4 mm Hg in the blood [58]. These data suggest that the benefits of salt reduction seen in patients who have prehypertension may not benefit patients on hypertensive therapy with calcium-channel blockers.

In addition to dietary modifications, engaging in regular aerobic exercise, such as brisk walking for at least 30 minutes a day or swimming most days of the week, is recommended by JNC7. It is estimated that such regular physical activity will result in approximately a 4- to 9-mm Hg fall in systolic blood pressure [59,60]. Regular aerobic exercise of mild-to-moderate intensity lowers blood pressure in patients who have essential hypertension [61,62]. Sedentary lifestyle increases risk for elevated blood pressure, whereas increased leisure time or occupational physical activity is associated with lower levels of blood pressure [63]. In a recent study, aerobic exercise was associated with a 4-mm Hg reduction in systolic and diastolic blood pressure [64]. The investigators found that although exercise alone was effective in reducing blood pressure, the addition of a behavioral weight loss regimen enhanced this effect. Weight loss was associated with a 7-mm Hg systolic and 5-mm Hg diastolic reduction in blood pressure. Animal studies have reported that exercise in rats that have hypertension results in widespread cardiac fibrosis, an important precursor to diastolic dysfunction and proarrhythmia [65]. One study reported that excessive and uncontrolled exercise in hypertensive animals can result in adverse cardiac remodeling and progression to heart failure [66]. The impact of exercise on blood pressure and heart failure is intriguing. Further studies are needed to determine the impact of well-defined exercise protocols at different levels of intensity in hypertension and heart failure.

JNC7 recommends regular physical activity to ensure weight loss and maintain weight loss. It recommends regular aerobic physical activity at least 30 minutes per day on most days of the week.

Despite JNC7 recommendations, realistically incorporating healthier lifestyles into everyday life has been difficult and not long lasting. An effective approach requires a system-wide approach to achieve long-lasting reductions in weight loss and blood pressure. Several strategies have been recommended that require buy-in from employers, insurers, managed care organizations, community groups, media outlets, and schools to facilitate necessary changes. Increasing pressure may be needed on food and restaurant industries to offer healthier low-salt products, not dissimilar to the trans fat ban in New York City. Public school systems should incorporate a curriculum on health issues and get rid of unhealthy meals on their menus and vending machines on their premises. The community at large should make available areas and programs to increase physical activity. Realistically, new federal legislation and policies may be required to achieve these necessary goals. The health care system should be updated to provide incentive to physicians and other care providers to institute effective dietary and lifestyle counseling. Only then would these physicians reorganize their clinical practice to provide preventive care.

Sleep apnea

Efforts to improve sleep apnea have been recommended by JNC7. In addition to weight loss, it emphasizes the importance of continuous positive airway pressure in lowering blood pressure and improving cardiac ischemia and symptoms of heart failure [67,68]. It does not recommend any specific class of blood pressure–reducing agents for patients with obstructive sleep apnea.

Pharmacotherapy

Although preventing heart failure is an important goal of JNC7 guidelines, the overall focus is on preventing cardiovascular morbidity and mortality. More than two thirds of individuals with elevated blood pressure have stage 2 hypertension (ie, systolic blood pressure > 160 mm Hg), which is not controlled by one drug and requires two or more blood pressure–reducing agents selected from different classes to achieve blood pressure goals (Fig. 5) [22,69–72]. In the Antihypertensive and Lipid-lowering Treatment to Prevent Heart Attack Trial (ALLHAT), only 30% of the overall cohort was controlled with one drug alone; approximately 60% required at least two antihypertensive agents to achieve blood pressure less than 140/90 mm Hg. In some patients who required lower blood goals or had substantially elevated blood pressure, three or more blood pressure–

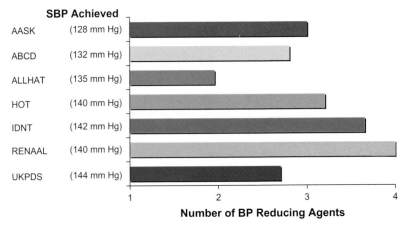

Fig. 5. Patients who have hypertension and multiple risk factors require multiple agents to achieve a systolic blood pressure goal. AASK, African American Study of Kidney Disease and Hypertension [111]; ABCD, appropriate blood pressure control in diabetes [112–114]; ALLHAT, Antihypertensive and Lipid-Lowering Treatment to Prevent Heart Attack Trial [75]; HOT, hypertension optimal treatment [22,112]; IDNT, Irbesartan Diabetic Nephropathy Trial [115]; RENAAL, Reduction of Endpoints in NIDDM With the Angiotensin II Antagonist Losartan [116]; UKPDS, UK Prospective Diabetes Study [112,117].

reducing medications may be required. Determining an appropriate antihypertensive regimen frequently consists of using several drugs in combination. One meta-analysis of randomized placebo-controlled trials of antihypertensive therapy reported that adequate blood pressure control decreases the incidence of heart failure by half [73].

Diuretic-based antihypertensive treatment regimens repeatedly have been reported to prevent heart failure in a wide range of target populations [74]. ACE inhibitors and beta-blockers also effectively prevent heart failure [16], whereas calcium-channel blockers and alpha-blockers are less effective in preventing heart failure syndrome [75]. Beta-blockers and ACE inhibitors as monotherapies are not superior to other antihypertensive drug classes in reducing all cardiovascular outcomes. In patients who have diabetes or other cardiovascular complications [76,77], ACE inhibitors have been most notable with respect to a reduction in the onset of heart failure and new-onset diabetes. Similarly, the angiotensin receptor blockers (ARBs) losartan [78] and irbesartan [79], when compared with placebo, significantly reduced the incidence of heart failure in patients who had type 2 diabetes mellitus and nephropathy.

Prevention of heart failure

Only thiazide diuretics have been shown to consistently prevent disease progression of heart failure associated with hypertension (Fig. 6). In the Systolic Hypertension in the Elderly study, patients with isolated systolic hypertension and a previous evidence of myocardial infarction who were treated with a diuretic-based treatment plan that lowered systolic blood pressure to less than 150 mm Hg experienced a 2% to 3% chance of developing heart failure over a 4-year period [20]. Patients treated with a placebo had an 8% to 10% chance of developing heart failure, however. In the ALLHAT, which was a double-blind, randomized clinical trial of 33,357 high-risk patients older than age 55 who had hypertension, the relative risks of heart failure (95% confidence intervals; P values) using amlodipine or lisinopril versus chlorthalidone were 1.35 (1.21–1.50; $P <$ .001) and 1.11 (0.99–1.24; $P = 0.09$), respectively. During year 1, the relative risks of amlodipine or lisinopril versus chlorthalidone were 2.22 (1.69–2.91; $P <$ .001) and 2.08 (1.58–2.74; $P < 0.001$), respectively; after year 1, the risks were 1.22 (1.08–1.38; $P = $ .001) and 0.96 (0.85–1.10; $P = $

0.58), respectively. These results suggested that thiazide diuretics are superior to calcium-channel blockers and, in the short term, to ACE inhibitors in preventing heart failure in individuals who have hypertension.

Left ventricular hypertrophy regresses with aggressive blood pressure reduction induced by sodium restriction, weight loss, and treatment with most antihypertensive medications except direct afterload-reducing agents, such as minoxidil and hydralazine [80,81]. One meta-analysis of 50 studies of left ventricular hypertophic regression conducted before 1996 reported that the most consistent reduction in left ventricular mass was associated with ACE inhibitors, intermediate benefits were achieved with calcium-channel blockers and diuretics, and the least reduction was achieved with beta-blockers [82]. In the VA Cooperative Monotherapy trial and the Treatment of Mild Hypertension study (TOMHS), however, diuretic therapy achieved the best reduction in left ventricular mass [83,84]. The more recent Losartan Intervention for Endpoint Reduction in Hypertension study reported that left ventricular hypertrophy as defined by electrocardiogram changes was significantly reduced with ARB losartan when compared with an atenolol-based regimen despite a comparable reduction in blood pressure [69].

One paradigm shift in the JNC7 report was that beta-blockers were no longer first-line agents in the management of hypertension. For more than three decades, these agents were recommended as first-line therapy in the management of hypertension; however, multiple prospective, randomized trials have reported that diuretic-based antihypertensive agents reduce risk of stroke and, to a lesser extent, the risk of myocardial infarction and cardiovascular morbidity [69,85–87]. The data with beta-blockers have been less robust [88], with no study demonstrating that their monotherapeutic usage is associated with a reduction in morbidity or mortality when compared with placebo. Only the Metoprolol Atherosclerosis Prevention in Hypertension study showed superiority of beta-blockers to diuretic therapy for the initial treatment of hypertension [89]. The British Medical Research Council trial in older adults reported that beta-blockers were ineffective [85]. When beta-blockers were added to diuretics, there was some blunting of the beneficial effects of the antihypertensive regimen [85,90].

More recently the Anglo–Scandinavian Cardiac Outcomes Trial-Blood Pressure Lowering

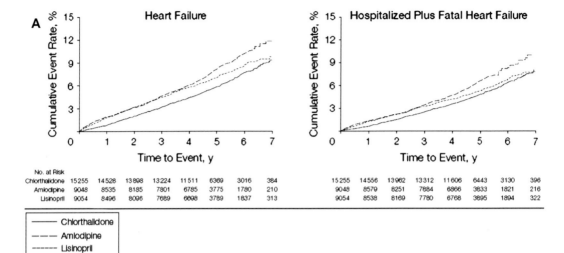

Fig. 6. (*A*) Cumulative event rates for heart failure and hospitalized plus fatal heart failure by treatment group. (*B*) Relative risks and 95% confidence intervals for lisinopril/chlorthalidone comparisons in prespecified subgroups. (*C*) Relative risks and 95% confidence intervals (CIs) for amlodipine/chlorthalidone comparisons in prespecified subgroups. (A–C *Modified from* ALLHAT Officers and Coordinators for the ALLHAT Collaborative Research Group. The Antihypertensive and Lipid-Lowering Treatment to Prevent Heart Attack Trial. Major outcomes in high-risk hypertensive patients randomized to ACE inhibitor or calcium channel blocker versus diuretic: the Antihypertensive and Lipid-Lowering Treatment to Prevent Heart Attack Trial (ALLHAT). JAMA 2002;288(23):2981–97; with permission.) (*D*) Relative risks for comparisons of amlodipine versus chlorthalidone and lisinopril versus chlorthalidone in blacks and nonblacks. (*E*) Heart failure rate for blacks and nonblacks, by treatment group. (D, E *Modified from* Wright JT Jr, Dunn JK, Cutler JA, et al. Outcomes in hypertensive black and nonblack patients treated with chlorthalidone, amlodipine, and lisinopril. JAMA 2005;293(13):1595–608; with permission.)

D

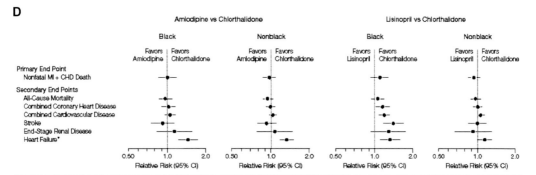

Scales are shown in natural logarithm. The proportional hazards assumption was violated for heart failure, so relative risks and 95% confidence intervals (CIs) were calculated using 2×2 tables. *Includes fatal, nonfatal hospitalized, and nonhospitalized treated. CHD indicates coronary heart disease; MI, myocardial infarction.

E

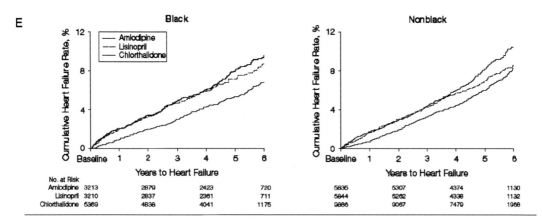

Fig. 6 (*continued*)

Arm study, which was composed of a cohort of 19,257 individuals who had hypertension and at least three other coronary risk factors but no clinically overt coronary heart disease, reported that atenolol-based treatment resulted in a 14% greater risk of coronary events and 23% greater risk of stroke when compared with an amlodipine-based regimen [86]. Pooled analyses have reported that beta-blockers reduce the risk of stroke by 16% to 22%, which is less superior to a 38% reduction by other antihypertensive agents for the same degree of blood pressure reduction [91]. In one meta-analysis of 13 randomized, controlled studies that involved approximately 105,000 patients, initial therapy with beta-blockers was associated with a 16% higher relative risk of stroke (95% confidence interval 4%–30%) compared with other blood pressure–reducing agents [87]. The best beta-blocker used for managing hypertension is atenolol. One meta-analysis reported that when compared with placebo, atenolol was no different in reducing all-cause or cardiovascular mortality,

and only a trend for reducing the incidence of stroke (Fig. 7) [92]. Unfortunately these data have resulted in all beta-blockers being painted with the same brush. Not all beta-blockers are the same, however, and as a class they represent a diverse group of drugs with disparate pharmacologic properties. They may block both β1- and β2-adrenergic receptors nonselectively or they may preferentially block the cardioselective β1 receptors.

Two promising beta-blockers in the management of hypertension are carvedilol [93] and nebivolol. Carvedilol has been shown to be efficacious in the management of heart failure and is a cardioselective agent with vasodilatory properties. The Glycemic Effects in Diabetes Mellitus: Carvedilol-Metoprolol Comparison in Hypertensives study demonstrated that carvedilol does not worsen glucose intolerance [94]. Similarly, nebivolol does not impair glucose tolerance [95]; it is cardioselective and vasodilating. The Study of the Effects of Nebivolol Intervention in Outcomes and

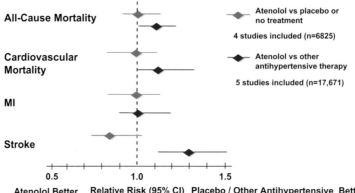

Fig. 7. β1-Selective atenolol and adverse outcomes in patients with HTN. Trials included in meta-analysis versus placebo: Treatment of Hypertension in Elderly Patients in Primary Care (HEP); Dutch Transitory Ischemic Attack Trial; Tenormin After Stroke and TIA (TEST); Medical Research Council Trial of Treatment of Hypertension in Older Adults (MRC Old). Trials included in meta-analysis versus other antihypertensive agent: MRC Old; UKPDS; European Lacidipine Study of Atherosclerosis (ELSA); Heart Attack Primary Prevention in Hypertension Trial (HAPPHY); Losartan Intervention for Endpoint Reduction Study (LIFE). (*Data from* Carlberg B, Samuelsson O, Lindholm LH. Atenolol in hypertension: is it a wise choice? Lancet 2004;364(9446):1684–89.)

Rehospitalization in Seniors demonstrated that nebivolol is well tolerated by older patients who have heart failure [96]. Although the use of beta-blockers in uncomplicated hypertension continues to wane, their use in patients who have heart failure continues to increase. Heart failure is a hyperadrenergic state with up-regulation of adrenergic receptors on the myocardium with long-term results in myocardial remodeling, cardiac fibrosis, and propensity for life-threatening ventricular arrhythmias. Beta-blockers probably protect the heart from deleterious effects of epinephrine and norepinephrine and remain the cornerstone of therapy in these patients. Hypertension in elderly persons is accompanied by decreased adrenergic responsiveness, decreased heart rate and cardiac output, and decreased arterial compliance. There is a paucity of data to support the use of beta-blockers in uncomplicated hypertension. In patients who have hypertension complicated by cardiac tachyarrhythmias, coronary artery disease, myocardial infarction, systolic heart failure, and hypertrophic cardiomyopathy, beta-blockers remain important therapeutic agents in the management of these conditions.

Before the results of ALLHAT were available, several researchers expected that lisinopril would be as efficacious—if not better—in preventing heart failure compared with chlorthalidone. Previous studies reported that ACE inhibitors are beneficial

in heart failure [97]. There is also a solid pharmacologic rationale to anticipate these results, because ACE inhibitors block the renin-angiotensin system, whereas diuretics stimulate this system. Despite this rationale, chlorthalidone was superior to lisinopril not only in preventing heart failure but also in preventing strokes and combined cardiovascular disease (Fig. 6B). The findings of increased risk of heart failure (statistically significant for total heart failure) are intriguing because the benefits of ACE inhibitors in heart failure are well documented.

Calcium-channel blockers seem to be particularly efficacious in African Americans with regard to monotherapy according to one meta-analysis. In this analysis they seemed to be efficacious in all stages of hypertension, including in patients with diastolic blood pressure more than 110 mm Hg [98]. The ultimate goal of antihypertensive therapy is to optimally protect target organs, however. The ALLHAT study demonstrated that diuretics were superior to calcium-channel blockers in lowering blood pressure and preventing heart failure in African Americans, as in the larger population (Fig. 6C–E) [99].

Systolic heart failure

The JNC7 discusses the American College of Cardiology/American Heart Association (ACC/AHA) guidelines for management of heart failure.

A

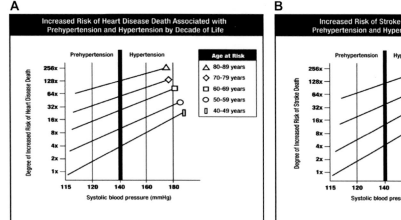

B

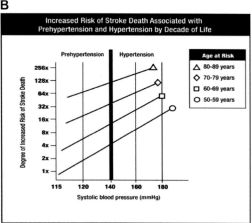

Fig. 8. The new high blood pressure guidelines classify persons with systolic blood pressures of 120 to 139 mm Hg or diastolic blood pressures of 80 to 89 mm Hg as prehypertensive. (*A*) The risk of heart disease death begins to rise at a systolic blood pressure of 115. For every 20-mm Hg increase above that, the risk of heart disease death doubles. The increase in risk occurs at every decade of life. (*B*) The risk of stroke death begins to rise at a systolic blood pressure of 115. For every 20-mm Hg increase above that, the risk of stroke death doubles. The increase in risk occurs at every decade of life. (*Data from* Prospective Studies Collaboration. Age-specific relevance of usual blood pressure to vascular mortality: a meta-analysis of individual data for one million adults in 61 prospective studies. Lancet 2002;360:1903–13. *From* National Heart, Lung, and Blood Institute. Media Kit for The Seventh Report of the Joint National Committee on Prevention, Detection, Evaluation, and Treatment of High Blood Pressure (JNC 7). Available at: http://www.nhlbi.nih.gov/guidelines/hypertension/media_kit.htm. Accessed September 27, 2007.)

The ACC/AHA guidelines have recommended that in patients with stage A heart failure (ie, patients at high risk for heart failure but with no clinical symptoms or signs of left ventricular dysfunction), treatment should include meticulous management of hyperlipidemia, hyperglycemia, and blood pressure. For patients at high risk of cardiovascular disease, ACE inhibitors may be appropriate because of their beneficial effects on survival [76,77]. The ALLHAT study suggested that preventing progression of heart failure may be achieved by the use of thiazide diuretics [75]. In ACC/AHA stage B heart failure (NYHA class I), which is defined as left ventricular dysfunction with an ejection fraction of less than 40%, it is recommended ACE inhibitors and beta-blockers be used. Aldosterone receptor blockers may be beneficial in selected patients, particularly after myocardial infarction [100–102]. In ACC/AHA stage C heart failure (NYHA class II-III), which is defined as the presence of left ventricular dysfunction with overt symptoms, the recommendations is to use ACE inhibitors and beta-blockers. Aldosterone receptor blockers may be beneficial in these patients [100–102]. Loop diuretics are useful in restoring euvolemia but can result in cardiorenal syndrome. In ACC/AHA stage D heart failure (NYHA class IV), the choice of blood pressure–reducing agents must be weighed to reflect the requirements of advanced care, such as inotropic drugs, biventricular pacemakers, automatic implantable defibrillators, and cardiac transplantation or right- and left-ventricular mechanical assist devices.

The JNC7 report classifies heart failure as a compelling indication (the compelling indication is managed in parallel with the blood pressure) for the use of diuretics, ACE inhibitors, beta-blockers, angiotensin-receptor blockers, and aldosterone antagonists. Calcium-channel blockers are not indicated in heart failure as a compelling indication because of the lack efficacy in these patients [103]. The basis of JNC7's recommendation for ACE inhibitors is the plethora of literature demonstrating the value of these agents in this setting [104–106]. Similarly, beta-blockers are recommended in heart failure because of clinical studies reporting the reduction in morbidity and mortality in patients with symptoms of heart failure [107–109]. Aldosterone receptor blockers are recommended because evidence suggests their use in late stage C heart failure (NYHA class III-IV) [101] and heart failure after myocardial infarction [102].

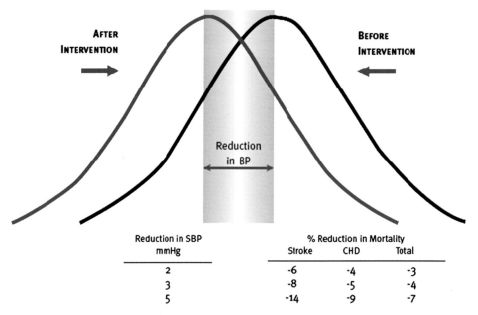

Reduction in SBP mmHg	% Reduction in Mortality		
	Stroke	CHD	Total
2	-6	-4	-3
3	-8	-5	-4
5	-14	-9	-7

BP, blood pressure; CHD, coronary heart disease; SBP, systolic blood pressure

Source: Whelton PK, et al. Primary prevention of hypertension: Clinical and public health advisory from The National High Blood Pressure Education Program. JAMA 2002;288:1882–8.

Fig. 9. Impact of reducing blood pressure on total mortality and mortality due to stroke and coronary heart disease. (*From* Whelton PK, He J, Appel LJ, et al. Primary prevention of hypertension: clinical and public health advisory from the National High Blood Pressure Education Program. JAMA 2002;288:1882–8; with permission.)

Although JNC7 does not specify blood pressure targets for patients who have heart failure, it recommends that low blood pressure may be desirable in patients. In most clinical trials of heart failure, systolic blood pressure was successfully reduced to the range of 110 to 130 mm Hg. One trial demonstrated the benefits of beta-blockade in patients with systolic blood pressure more than 85 mm Hg, which suggested that low blood pressure is easily tolerated by these patients [108]. A recent study suggested that antihypertensive therapy may be intensified when systolic blood pressure is not under control in elderly persons—at least until diastolic blood pressure reaches 55 mm Hg—unless coronary artery disease is also present, in which case diastolic blood pressure probably should not be lowered to less than 70 mm Hg to allow coronary perfusion during diastole [110].

designed not only to reduce the incidence of heart failure but also prevent other target end-organ damage and reduce overall cardiovascular morbidity and mortality. The emphasis of these recommendations is to reduce systolic blood pressure, because the risk of mortality caused by heart disease and stroke doubles for every 20-mm Hg increase in systolic blood pressure (Fig. 8). Reducing systolic blood pressure even by 2 mm Hg reduces overall mortality by 3%; reducing it by 5 mm Hg reduces stroke-related mortality by 14%, coronary heart disease–related mortality by 9%, and overall mortality by 7% (Fig. 9). Practitioners are encouraged to use a combination of lifestyle changes and pharmacotherapy to achieve systolic blood pressure goals and consider the use of thiazide diuretics as first-line therapy to achieve the ultimate goal of reducing end-organ damage.

Summary

If the recommendations of JNC7 are implemented, the incidence of heart failure should continue to decline. These recommendations are

References

[1] Levy D, et al. The progression from hypertension to congestive heart failure. JAMA 1996;275(20): 1557–62.

[2] Vasan RS, et al. Residual lifetime risk for developing hypertension in middle-aged women and men: the Framingham Heart Study. JAMA 2002; 287(8):1003–10.

[3] Levy D, et al. Long-term trends in the incidence of and survival with heart failure. N Engl J Med 2002; 347(18):1397–402.

[4] Rosamond W, et al. Heart disease and stroke statistics: 2007 update. a report from the American Heart Association Statistics Committee and Stroke Statistics Subcommittee. Circulation 2007;115(5): e69–171.

[5] Haider AW, et al. Systolic blood pressure, diastolic blood pressure, and pulse pressure as predictors of risk for congestive heart failure in the Framingham Heart Study. Ann Intern Med 2003;138(1):10–6.

[6] Chae CU, et al. Increased pulse pressure and risk of heart failure in the elderly. JAMA 1999;281(7): 634–9.

[7] Vaccarino V, et al. Pulse pressure and risk of cardiovascular events in the systolic hypertension in the elderly program. Am J Cardiol 2001;88(9): 980–6.

[8] Vaccarino V, Holford TR, Krumholz HM. Pulse pressure and risk for myocardial infarction and heart failure in the elderly. J Am Coll Cardiol 2000;36(1):130–8.

[9] Kannel WB, et al. Role of blood pressure in the development of congestive heart failure: The Framingham study. N Engl J Med 1972;287(16):781–7.

[10] Cooper RS, et al. Left ventricular hypertrophy is associated with worse survival independent of ventricular function and number of coronary arteries severely narrowed. Am J Cardiol 1990;65(7):441–5.

[11] Ghali JK, et al. The prognostic role of left ventricular hypertrophy in patients with or without coronary artery disease. Ann Intern Med 1992;117(10): 831–6.

[12] Levy D, et al. Prognostic implications of echocardiographically determined left ventricular mass in the Framingham Heart Study. N Engl J Med 1990;322(22):1561–6.

[13] Senni M, et al. Congestive heart failure in the community: a study of all incident cases in Olmsted County, Minnesota, in 1991. Circulation 1998; 98(21):2282–9.

[14] McMurray J, et al. Clinical features and contemporary management of patients with low and preserved ejection fraction heart failure: baseline characteristics of patients in the Candesartan in Heart failure-Assessment of Reduction in Mortality and Morbidity (CHARM) programme. Eur J Heart Fail 2003;5(3):261–70.

[15] Senni M, Redfield MM. Heart failure with preserved systolic function: a different natural history? J Am Coll Cardiol 2001;38(5):1277–82.

[16] Chobanian AV, et al. The seventh report of the Joint National Committee on prevention, detection, evaluation, and treatment of high blood pressure: the JNC 7 report. JAMA 2003;289(19): 2560–72.

[17] Wilhelmsen L, et al. Heart failure in the general population of men: morbidity, risk factors and prognosis. J Intern Med 2001;249(3):253–61.

[18] Effects of treatment on morbidity in hypertension. II. Results in patients with diastolic blood pressure averaging 90 through 114 mm Hg. JAMA 1970; 213(7):1143–52.

[19] Izzo JL Jr, Gradman AH. Mechanisms and management of hypertensive heart disease: from left ventricular hypertrophy to heart failure. Med Clin North Am 2004;88(5):1257–71.

[20] Kostis JB, et al. Prevention of heart failure by antihypertensive drug treatment in older persons with isolated systolic hypertension: SHEP Cooperative Research Group. JAMA 1997;278(3):212–6.

[21] Baker DW. Prevention of heart failure. J Card Fail 2002;8(5):333–46.

[22] Hansson L, et al. Effects of intensive blood-pressure lowering and low-dose aspirin in patients with hypertension: principal results of the hypertension optimal treatment (HOT) randomised trial. HOT Study Group. Lancet 1998;351(9118): 1755–62.

[23] UK Prospective Diabetes Study Group. Tight blood pressure control and risk of macrovascular and microvascular complications in type 2 diabetes: UKPDS 38. BMJ 1998;317(7160):703–13.

[24] Cohn JN, Johnson G. Heart failure with normal ejection fraction: the V-HeFT Study. Veterans Administration Cooperative Study Group. Circulation 1990;81(2 Suppl):III48–53.

[25] Dougherty AH, et al. Congestive heart failure with normal systolic function. Am J Cardiol 1984;54(7): 778–82.

[26] Echeverria HH, et al. Congestive heart failure: echocardiographic insights. Am J Med 1983;75(5): 750–5.

[27] Soufer R, et al. Intact systolic left ventricular function in clinical congestive heart failure. Am J Cardiol 1985;55(8):1032–6.

[28] Bhatia RS, et al. Outcome of heart failure with preserved ejection fraction in a population-based study. N Engl J Med 2006;355(3): 260–9.

[29] Kitzman DW, et al. Pathophysiological characterization of isolated diastolic heart failure in comparison to systolic heart failure. JAMA 2002;288(17): 2144–50.

[30] Drukteinis JS, Roman MJ, Fabsitz RR, et al. Cardiac and systemic hemodynamic characteristics of hypertension and prehypertension in adolescents and young adults: the Strong Heart Study. Circulation 2007;115:221–7.

[31] Oki T, et al. Left ventricular diastolic properties of hypertensive patients measured by pulsed tissue Doppler imaging. J Am Soc Echocardiogr 1998; 11(12):1106–12.

[32] Ahn J, et al. Cardiac structural and functional responses to salt loading in SHR. Am J Physiol Heart Circ Physiol 2004;287(2):H767–72.

[33] Coca A, De la Sierra A. Salt sensitivity and left ventricular hypertrophy. Adv Exp Med Biol 1997; 432:91–101.

[34] Dahl LK, et al. Effects of chronic excess salt ingestion: modification of experimental hypertension in the rat by variations in the diet. Circ Res 1968; 22(1):11–8.

[35] Musiari L, et al. Early abnormalities in left ventricular diastolic function of sodium-sensitive hypertensive patients. J Hum Hypertens 1999;13(10):711–6.

[36] He FJ, MacGregor GA. Effect of longer-term modest salt reduction on blood pressure. Cochrane Database Syst Rev 2004;3:CD004937.

[37] He FJ, Markandu ND, MacGregor GA. Modest salt reduction lowers blood pressure in isolated systolic hypertension and combined hypertension. Hypertension 2005;46(1):66–70.

[38] Sacks FM, et al. Effects on blood pressure of reduced dietary sodium and the Dietary Approaches to Stop Hypertension (DASH) diet: DASH-Sodium Collaborative Research Group. N Engl J Med 2001;344(1):3–10.

[39] Kupari M, Koskinen P, Virolainen J. Correlates of left ventricular mass in a population sample aged 36 to 37 years: focus on lifestyle and salt intake. Circulation 1994;89(3):1041–50.

[40] Messerli FH, Schmieder RE, Weir MR. Salt: a perpetrator of hypertensive target organ disease? Arch Intern Med 1997;157(21):2449–52.

[41] Schmieder RE, et al. Dietary salt intake: a determinant of cardiac involvement in essential hypertension. Circulation 1988;78(4):951–6.

[42] Schmieder RE, et al. Sodium intake modulates left ventricular hypertrophy in essential hypertension. J Hypertens Suppl 1988;6(4):S148–50.

[43] Langenfeld MR, et al. Impact of dietary sodium intake on left ventricular diastolic filling in early essential hypertension. Eur Heart J 1998;19(6):951–8.

[44] Svetkey LP. Management of prehypertension. Hypertension 2005;45(6):1056–61.

[45] Appel LJ, et al. Effects of comprehensive lifestyle modification on blood pressure control: main results of the PREMIER clinical trial. JAMA 2003; 289(16):2083–93.

[46] Elmer PJ, et al. Effects of comprehensive lifestyle modification on diet, weight, physical fitness, and blood pressure control: 18-month results of a randomized trial. Ann Intern Med 2006;144(7):485–95.

[47] Bagrov AY, Lakatta EG. The dietary sodium-blood pressure plot "stiffens." Hypertension 2004; 44(1):22–4.

[48] Appel LJ, et al. A clinical trial of the effects of dietary patterns on blood pressure: DASH Collaborative Research Group. N Engl J Med 1997;336(16): 1117–24.

[49] He FJ, MacGregor GA. How far should salt intake be reduced? Hypertension 2003;42(6):1093–9.

[50] Erwteman TM, et al. Beta blockade, diuretics, and salt restriction for the management of mild hypertension: a randomised double blind trial. Br Med J (Clin Res Ed) 1984;289(6442):406–9.

[51] Suppa G, et al. Effects of a low-sodium high-potassium salt in hypertensive patients treated with metoprolol: a multicentre study. J Hypertens 1988;6(10):787–90.

[52] Carney SL, et al. Effect of dietary sodium restriction on patients receiving antihypertensive medication. Clin Exp Hypertens A 1984;6(6):1095–105.

[53] Hollenberg NK, et al. Sodium intake and renal responses to captopril in normal man and in essential hypertension. Kidney Int 1981;20(2):240–5.

[54] MacGregor GA, et al. Moderate sodium restriction with angiotensin converting enzyme inhibitor in essential hypertension: a double blind study. Br Med J (Clin Res Ed) 1987;294(6571):531–4.

[55] Kristinsson A, et al. Additive effects of moderate dietary salt reduction and captopril in hypertension. Acta Med Scand 1988;223(2):133–7.

[56] Cappuccio FP, Markandu ND, MacGregor GA. Calcium antagonists and sodium balance: effect of changes in sodium intake and of the addition of a thiazide diuretic on the blood pressure lowering effect of nifedipine. J Cardiovasc Pharmacol 1987; 10(Suppl 10):S57–61.

[57] MacGregor GA, Cappuccio FP, Markandu ND. Sodium intake, high blood pressure, and calcium channel blockers. Am J Med 1987;82(3B):16–22.

[58] Morgan T, Anderson A. Interaction of slow-channel calcium blocking drugs with sodium restriction, diuretics and angiotensin converting enzyme inhibitors. J Hypertens Suppl 1988;6(4):S652–4.

[59] Kelley GA, Kelley KS. Progressive resistance exercise and resting blood pressure: a meta-analysis of randomized controlled trials. Hypertension 2000; 35(3):838–43.

[60] Whelton SP, et al. Effect of aerobic exercise on blood pressure: a meta-analysis of randomized, controlled trials. Ann Intern Med 2002;136(7):493–503.

[61] Dengel DR, et al. Improvements in blood pressure, glucose metabolism, and lipoprotein lipids after aerobic exercise plus weight loss in obese, hypertensive middle-aged men. Metabolism 1998;47(9): 1075–82.

[62] Kokkinos PF, et al. Effects of regular exercise on blood pressure and left ventricular hypertrophy in African-American men with severe hypertension. N Engl J Med 1995;333(22):1462–7.

[63] World Hypertension League. Physical exercise in the management of hypertension: a consensus statement by the World Hypertension League. J Hypertens 1991;9(3):283–7.

[64] Blumenthal JA, et al. Exercise and weight loss reduce blood pressure in men and women with mild

hypertension: effects on cardiovascular, metabolic, and hemodynamic functioning. Arch Intern Med 2000;160(13):1947–58.

[65] Sarma S, Schulze PC. Exercise as a physiologic intervention to counteract hypertension: can a good idea go bad? Hypertension 2007;50(2):294–6.

[66] Piepoli MF, et al. Exercise training meta-analysis of trials in patients with chronic heart failure (ExTraMATCH). BMJ 2004;328(7433):189–96.

[67] Dart RA, et al. The association of hypertension and secondary cardiovascular disease with sleep-disordered breathing. Chest 2003;123(1):244–60.

[68] Wolk R, Kara T, Somers VK. Sleep-disordered breathing and cardiovascular disease. Circulation 2003;108(1):9–12.

[69] Dahlof B, et al. Cardiovascular morbidity and mortality in the Losartan Intervention For Endpoint reduction in hypertension study (LIFE): a randomised trial against atenolol. Lancet 2002;359(9311):995–1003.

[70] Materson BJ, et al. Single-drug therapy for hypertension in men: a comparison of six antihypertensive agents with placebo. The Department of Veterans Affairs Cooperative Study Group on Antihypertensive Agents. N Engl J Med 1993;328(13):914–21.

[71] Cushman WC, et al. Success and predictors of blood pressure control in diverse North American settings: the antihypertensive and lipid-lowering treatment to prevent heart attack trial (ALLHAT). J Clin Hypertens (Greenwich) 2002;4(6):393–404.

[72] Black HR, et al. Principal results of the controlled onset verapamil investigation of cardiovascular end points (CONVINCE) trial. JAMA 2003;289(16):2073–82.

[73] Moser M, Hebert PR. Prevention of disease progression, left ventricular hypertrophy and congestive heart failure in hypertension treatment trials. J Am Coll Cardiol 1996;27(5):1214–8.

[74] Staessen JA, Wang JG, Thijs L. Cardiovascular protection and blood pressure reduction: a meta-analysis. Lancet 2001;358(9290):1305–15.

[75] ALLHAT investigators. Major outcomes in high-risk hypertensive patients randomized to angiotensin-converting enzyme inhibitor or calcium channel blocker vs diuretic: the antihypertensive and lipid-lowering treatment to prevent heart attack trial (ALLHAT). JAMA 2002;288(23):2981–97.

[76] Fox KM. Efficacy of perindopril in reduction of cardiovascular events among patients with stable coronary artery disease: randomised, double-blind, placebo-controlled, multicentre trial (the EUROPA study). Lancet 2003;362(9386):782–8.

[77] Yusuf S, et al. Effects of an angiotensin-converting-enzyme inhibitor, ramipril, on cardiovascular events in high-risk patients: the Heart Outcomes Prevention Evaluation Study Investigators. N Engl J Med 2000;342(3):145–53.

[78] Brenner BM, et al. Effects of losartan on renal and cardiovascular outcomes in patients with type 2 diabetes and nephropathy. N Engl J Med 2001;345(12):861–9.

[79] Berl T, et al. Cardiovascular outcomes in the Irbesartan Diabetic Nephropathy Trial of patients with type 2 diabetes and overt nephropathy. Ann Intern Med 2003;138(7):542–9.

[80] Kjeldsen SE, et al. Effects of losartan on cardiovascular morbidity and mortality in patients with isolated systolic hypertension and left ventricular hypertrophy: a Losartan Intervention for Endpoint Reduction (LIFE) substudy. JAMA 2002;288(12):1491–8.

[81] The sixth report of the Joint National Committee on prevention, detection, evaluation, and treatment of high blood pressure. Arch Intern Med 1997;157(21):2413–46.

[82] Schmieder RE, et al. Update on reversal of left ventricular hypertrophy in essential hypertension (a meta-analysis of all randomized double-blind studies until December 1996). Nephrol Dial Transplant 1998;13(3):564–9.

[83] Liebson PR, et al. Comparison of five antihypertensive monotherapies and placebo for change in left ventricular mass in patients receiving nutritional-hygienic therapy in the Treatment of Mild Hypertension Study (TOMHS). Circulation 1995;91(3):698–706.

[84] Gottdiener JS, et al. Effect of single-drug therapy on reduction of left ventricular mass in mild to moderate hypertension: comparison of six antihypertensive agents. The Department of Veterans Affairs Cooperative Study Group on Antihypertensive Agents. Circulation 1997;95(8):2007–14.

[85] Medical Research Council trial of treatment of hypertension in older adults: principal results. MRC Working Party. BMJ 1992;304(6824):405–12.

[86] Dahlof B, et al. Prevention of cardiovascular events with an antihypertensive regimen of amlodipine adding perindopril as required versus atenolol adding bendroflumethiazide as required, in the Anglo-Scandinavian Cardiac Outcomes Trial-Blood Pressure Lowering Arm (ASCOT-BPLA): a multicentre randomised controlled trial. Lancet 2005;366(9489):895–906.

[87] Lindholm LH, Carlberg B, Samuelsson O. Should beta blockers remain first choice in the treatment of primary hypertension? A meta-analysis. Lancet 2005;366(9496):1545–53.

[88] Messerli FH, Grossman E, Goldbourt U. Are beta-blockers efficacious as first-line therapy for hypertension in the elderly? A systematic review. JAMA 1998;279(23):1903–7.

[89] Wikstrand J, et al. Primary prevention with metoprolol in patients with hypertension: mortality

results from the MAPHY study. JAMA 1988; 259(13):1976–82.

[90] Lever AF, Brennan PJ. MRC trial of treatment in elderly hypertensives. Clin Exp Hypertens 1993; 15(6):941–52.

[91] Collins R, et al. Blood pressure, stroke, and coronary heart disease. Part 2. Short-term reductions in blood pressure: overview of randomised drug trials in their epidemiological context. Lancet 1990; 335(8693):827–38.

[92] Carlberg B, Samuelsson O, Lindholm LH. Atenolol in hypertension: is it a wise choice? Lancet 2004;364(9446):1684–9.

[93] Weber MA, et al. Controlled-release carvedilol in the treatment of essential hypertension. Am J Cardiol 2006;98(7A):32L–8L.

[94] Bakris GL, et al. Metabolic effects of carvedilol vs metoprolol in patients with type 2 diabetes mellitus and hypertension: a randomized controlled trial. JAMA 2004;292(18):2227–36.

[95] Peter P, et al. Effect of treatment with nebivolol on parameters of oxidative stress in type 2 diabetics with mild to moderate hypertension. J Clin Pharm Ther 2006;31(2):153–9.

[96] Flather MD, et al. Randomized trial to determine the effect of nebivolol on mortality and cardiovascular hospital admission in elderly patients with heart failure (SENIORS). Eur Heart J 2005;26(3): 215–25.

[97] SOLVD investigators. Effect of enalapril on mortality and the development of heart failure in asymptomatic patients with reduced left ventricular ejection fractions: the SOLVD Investigators. N Engl J Med 1992;327(10):685–91.

[98] Brewster LM, van Montfrans GA, Kleijnen J, et al. Antihypertensive drug therapy in black patients. Ann Intern Med 2004;141(8):614–27.

[99] Wright JT Jr, et al. Outcomes in hypertensive black and nonblack patients treated with chlorthalidone, amlodipine, and lisinopril. JAMA 2005;293(13): 1595–608.

[100] Baliga RR, et al. Spironolactone treatment and clinical outcomes in patients with systolic dysfunction and mild heart failure symptoms: a retrospective analysis. J Card Fail 2006;12(4):250–6.

[101] Pitt B, et al. The effect of spironolactone on morbidity and mortality in patients with severe heart failure: Randomized Aldactone Evaluation Study Investigators. N Engl J Med 1999;341(10): 709–17.

[102] Pitt B, et al. Eplerenone, a selective aldosterone blocker, in patients with left ventricular dysfunction after myocardial infarction. N Engl J Med 2003;348(14):1309–21.

[103] Packer M, et al. Effect of amlodipine on morbidity and mortality in severe chronic heart failure: Prospective Randomized Amlodipine Survival Evaluation Study Group. N Engl J Med 1996;335(15): 1107–14.

[104] SOLVD investigators. Effect of enalapril on survival in patients with reduced left ventricular ejection fractions and congestive heart failure: the SOLVD investigators. N Engl J Med 1991;325(5): 293–302.

[105] AIRE investigators. Effect of ramipril on mortality and morbidity of survivors of acute myocardial infarction with clinical evidence of heart failure: the Acute Infarction Ramipril Efficacy (AIRE) study investigators. Lancet 1993;342(8875):821–8.

[106] Kober L, et al. A clinical trial of the angiotensin-converting-enzyme inhibitor trandolapril in patients with left ventricular dysfunction after myocardial infarction: Trandolapril Cardiac Evaluation (TRACE) Study Group. N Engl J Med 1995; 333(25):1670–6.

[107] MERIT-HF study group. Effect of metoprolol CR/XL in chronic heart failure: Metoprolol CR/XL Randomised Intervention Trial in Congestive Heart Failure (MERIT-HF). Lancet 1999; 353(9169):2001–7.

[108] Packer M, et al. Effect of carvedilol on survival in severe chronic heart failure. N Engl J Med 2001; 344(22):1651–8.

[109] CIBIS study group. The Cardiac Insufficiency Bisoprolol Study II (CIBIS-II): a randomised trial. Lancet 1999;353(9146):9–13.

[110] Fagard R, Staessen JA, et al. On-treatment diastolic blood pressure and prognosis in systolic hypertension. 2007;167(17):1884–91.

[111] Wright JT Jr, et al. Effect of blood pressure lowering and antihypertensive drug class on progression of hypertensive kidney disease: results from the AASK trial. JAMA 2002;288(19):2421–31.

[112] Bakris GL. Maximizing cardiorenal benefit in the management of hypertension: achieve blood pressure goals. J Clin Hypertens (Greenwich) 1999; 1(2):141–7.

[113] Estacio RO, et al. The effect of nisoldipine as compared with enalapril on cardiovascular outcomes in patients with non-insulin-dependent diabetes and hypertension. N Engl J Med 1998;338(10):645–52.

[114] Estacio RO, et al. Effect of blood pressure control on diabetic microvascular complications in patients with hypertension and type 2 diabetes. Diabetes Care 2000;23(Suppl 2):B54–64.

[115] Lewis EJ, et al. Renoprotective effect of the angiotensin-receptor antagonist irbesartan in patients with nephropathy due to type 2 diabetes. N Engl J Med 2001;345(12):851–60.

[116] Bakris GL, et al. Effects of blood pressure level on progression of diabetic nephropathy: results from the RENAAL study. Arch Intern Med 2003; 163(13):1555–65.

[117] UK Prospective Diabetes Study Group. Efficacy of atenolol and captopril in reducing risk of macrovascular and microvascular complications in type 2 diabetes: UKPDS 39. BMJ 1998;317(7160): 713–20.

ELSEVIER
SAUNDERS

Cardiol Clin 25 (2007) 523–538

Heart Failure in the Diabetic Patient

David S.H. Bell, MB, FACP, FACE

University of Alabama Medical School, Birmingham, AL, USA

The number of patients with diabetes mellitus continues to rise in industrial societies owing mainly to changes in lifestyle (excessive calorie and fat intake and decreased physical activity). It is estimated that worldwide the number of affected adults will exceed 200 million within the next ten years. Of these diabetic subjects, 75% will die of cardiovascular disease and two thirds of these of cardiac disease [1]. Diabetes is a cardiac equivalent; a person with diabetes has greater than a 20% chance of experiencing a cardiac event within the next ten years, with the actual risk being 36% [2]. This risk places the type 2 diabetic subject in the same category as a patient with peripheral vascular disease or cerebrovascular disease or a patient who has an abdominal aortic aneurysm. A diabetic patient without known coronary artery disease has as much chance of having a myocardial infarct as a non-diabetic patient who has already had one [3]; therefore, there is no such thing as primary prevention of heart disease in the type 2 diabetic patient. For these patients, the goals for controlling cardiac risk factors are those of secondary prevention.

When a diabetic patient has a myocardial infarction, the rates of complications and mortality are twofold higher than in the non-diabetic patient, and the most common cause of heart failure (HF) following a myocardial infarction is diabetes [4,5]. The increased risk of HF in the post–myocardial infarction diabetic patient is not due solely to more extensive and distal coronary artery disease but also to hypertension/ventricular hypertrophy and diabetic cardiomyopathy.

The cardiotoxic triad of coronary artery disease, hypertension/ventricular hypertrophy, and diabetic cardiomyopathy also leads to decreased ventricular function in chronic and acute situations. Decreased ventricular function stimulates the renin-angiotensin (RAS) and the sympathetic nervous systems (SNS) which, in turn, leads to further myocardial damage and if untreated results in myocardial remodeling, arrhythmias, pump failure, and death.

It is not surprising that more than one third of type 2 diabetic patients die of HF, that diabetes is associated with a twofold to fivefold increase in the risk of HF, that HF is the most common diagnosis for admission to hospital for the diabetic patient, and that 44% of patients admitted to US hospitals with HF have diabetes [6–8].

In this review the extent of the increased rate of HF in the diabetic patient is examined, along with the possible causes for this increase and the poor prognosis associated with HF in the diabetic patient. Also reviewed are the therapies that are available for the treatment of diabetic HF and whether intensifying the use of these therapies might improve the worsened clinical outcomes for the patient who has diabetes.

Epidemiology of diabetic heart failure

The Framingham Heart Study showed that the prevalence of HF was twice as high in diabetic men and five times as high in diabetic women aged between 45 and 74 years when compared with age-matched controls [6]. Over age 65 years, the association became even stronger, with a fourfold higher prevalence in diabetic males and an eightfold higher prevalence in diabetic females [6]. In addition, the link between diabetes and HF grew stronger when patients with known ischemic heart disease were excluded [9,10].

E-mail address: dshbell@yahoo.com

In a health maintenance organization study of almost 10,000 type 2 diabetic patients, 12% had documented HF, and an analysis of this group showed that older age, longer duration of diabetes, insulin use, and a lower body mass index were independent risk factors [11]. Prospectively, in diabetic subjects who initially were without HF, HF developed at a rate of 3.3% per year [11]. Independent risk factors for the development of HF in this group were, once again, older age, longer duration of diabetes, use of insulin, and a lower body mass index but also surprisingly a lower HbA_{1c}. The paradoxical finding that a lower HbA_{1c} was associated with a greater incidence of HF could be explained by the increased likelihood that a patient with new-onset HF was more likely to have HbA_{1c} testing [11].

In a longitudinal study of elderly nursing home residents initially without a diagnosis of HF, HF developed over the next 43 months in 39% of those with diabetes and 23% of those without diabetes [12]. A cross-sectional study of an elderly Italian population with HF showed a 30% prevalence of diabetes [13]. The United Kingdom Prospective Diabetes Study, the largest study of type 2 diabetes ever performed, showed that the prevalence of HF in a group of newly diagnosed type 2 diabetic subjects was proportional to the HbA_{1c} level without an upper or a lower threshold [14]. Also in this study for every 1% increase in the HbA_{1c} level, there was a 16% increased risk of hospitalization for worsening HF or death [14].

Of patients requiring hospitalization for HF in the United States, 44% have diabetes, a percentage that seems to be increasing with time [15]. In the year 2000, patients with diabetes accounted for 38% of admissions with HF to an Alabama tertiary care hospital, which was similar to a statewide 33.6% of admissions with HF having diabetes [16].

There is also an increased incidence of diabetes in HF patients who, at the onset of HF, are euglycemic. In a 3-year prospective study of nondiabetic HF subjects, diabetes developed in 29% of HF patients compared with 18% of age- and gender-matched controls, and HF was shown to be an independent risk factor for the development of diabetes [13]. In studies of patients with idiopathic dilated cardiomyopathy (IDCM), the prevalence of diabetes was 60% to 100% higher than in a control population [17,18].

The underlying cause of the increased prevalence of diabetes in HF patients is likely to be an increase in insulin resistance caused by the increased SNS activity that is associated with HF. Insulin resistance has also been well documented in an IDCM population, and improvement in insulin resistance was demonstrated when an exercise program was initiated [19]. Almost half of an IDCM group who at onset were not known to have diabetes had increased insulin resistance when compared with matched controls, and when those subjects with known diabetes were included in the analysis 59% were shown to be insulin resistant [20]. IDCM patients are more insulin resistant than are patients with coronary artery disease as evidenced by elevated proinsulin levels in stored blood samples collected as much as 20 years before the clinical manifestations of IDCM appear [21,22]. Similarly, in a prospective study of Swedish patients, insulin resistance was independently associated with the development of HF [23].

In large-scale clinical HF trials, the percentage of diabetic patients is much lower than has been documented in the general population with HF. In the Cooperative North Scandinavian Enalapril Survival Study, only 23% of patients had diabetes, and in the Study of Left Ventricular Dysfunction (SOLVD), 25% had diabetes [24,25]. Diabetes also accounted for only 20% of subjects in the Vasodilation Heart Failure Trial II and the ATLAS (Assessment of Treatment with Lisinopril and Survival) study and 27% of subjects in RESOLVD (Randomized Evaluation for Strategies of Left Ventricular Dysfunction) [25–27]. In the CIBIS-II and BEST studies in which bucindolol was investigated in HF, only 11.8% and 35.6% of subjects had diabetes, respectively, and in MERIT-HF in which metoprolol was used for therapy of HF, only 24.7% of patients had diabetes [28–30]. In studies of the combined alpha- and beta-blocker carvedilol in HF, the ANZ, US Carvedilol, and COPERNICUS trials, 19.3%, 28.5%, and 25.7% of subjects had diabetes, respectively [31–33]. The misrepresentation of diabetic patients in HF trials attests to the desire of the sponsors to eliminate or minimize comorbidities and therefore lower adverse events. Unfortunately, when these drugs are used in the "real world," comorbidities can neither be minimized nor eliminated.

The prognosis for the diabetic patient with HF is worse than it is for the non-diabetic HF patient. In the SOLVD and RESOLVD trials, diabetes was an independent risk factor for mortality [25,27]. In the Diabetes Insulin Glucose in Acute Myocardial Infarction study, HF accounted for

66% of deaths in the year following the first myocardial infarction [34]. In the CARE study, a prospective post myocardial infarction study, the presence of diabetes increased the incidence of HF and death, and in a meta-analysis of diabetic subjects with HF treated with angiotensin-converting enzyme (ACE) inhibitors, the mortality rate was 11.5% per year [5,35]. When untreated and even partially treated, the prognosis for the diabetic subject with HF is worse than it is for the subject with non-diabetic HF [36]. The poor prognosis for the diabetic patient with HF might be related to the presence of insulin resistance. When the cause of HF was mechanical and due to mitral or aortic valve disease and not to myocardial ischemia, insulin resistance was associated with worsened outcomes that were independent of all other variables, including maximum oxygen consumption (VO_{2max}) and the severity of the HF [37].

Etiology of diabetic heart failure

Although it is clear that there is an association between diabetes and HF and a worse prognosis for the diabetic HF patient, the pathophysiologic explanation for these associations is less clear. The most likely explanation is the cardiotoxic triad of diabetic cardiomyopathy, coronary artery disease, and hypertension/ventricular hypertrophy [38]; however, the additions to the cardiotoxic triad of altered gene expression and autonomic dysfunction also have a significant role in the development and progression of diabetic HF [38].

The cardiotoxic triad

Cardiac function is impaired by the coexistence of myocardial ischemia, hypertension/ventricular hypertrophy, and a specific diabetic cardiomyopathy. Cooperatively and independently these three conditions contribute to anatomic, physiologic, and biochemical alterations in the myocardiocyte. Laboratory studies supported by clinical studies suggest that these overlapping etiologies have a major role in the development of HF in the diabetic patient.

Diabetic cardiomyopathy

The basic reason for the increased prevalence of HF in the diabetic patient is the presence of a distinct diabetic cardiomyopathy that pathologically is characterized by cardiomyocellular hypertrophy and fibrosis [39]. At a physiologic level, diabetic cardiomyopathy is associated with decreased myocardial mechanical function and electrophysiologic abnormalities. At a cellular level, it is associated with defects in subcellular organelles and down-regulation of catecholamine receptors due to chronically elevated catecholamine levels which occur in both the type 2 diabetic and insulin resistant patient but not in the type 1 diabetic patient [40,41]. Also, in animal models with the onset of hyperglycemia, changes in myocardial calcium transportation and alterations in contractile proteins occur, both of which lead to systolic and diastolic dysfunction that worsens as the collagen content of the myocardium increases [42–44].

Using a 1995 nationwide inpatient sample, a case-control study of patients discharged from the hospital with a diagnosis of idiopathic cardiomyopathy, it was determined that among subjects with this diagnosis there was a significant 75% increase in the prevalence of diabetes [17]. Also, there was an increased prevalence of idiopathic cardiomyopathy of 7.6 cases per 1000 discharged diabetic patients, which approached the 9.4 cases per 1000 discharged patients for diabetes-related lower-extremity amputations [17].

Investigating for early diastolic dysfunction in the diabetic patient through the use of sophisticated techniques such as tissue Doppler imaging has demonstrated that it is present at an early stage of diabetes. Rather than looking at blood flow, tissue Doppler imaging looks at the mitral annulus anatomically and shows a lesser pre-load dependent and a more linear expression of diastolic dysfunction than the more traditional echocardiographic methods of assessing diastolic dysfunction [45]. For example, a study of 80 children and adolescents with type 1 diabetes revealed evidence of left ventricular structural and filling abnormalities in a comparison with age-matched controls [46]. In addition, these abnormalities were more common in girls, which matched the findings of the Framingham Study in which the risk for congestive heart failure (CHF) was greater in women [6]. In adult diabetic subjects in Olmstead County, Minnesota, the prevalence of diastolic dysfunction was 52% and in Quebec 60% [44,47]. Using the ejection fraction as the sole measure of systolic function does not detect subtle systolic dysfunction. More sophisticated echocardiographic techniques such as peak strain and strain rate in a control-matched study demonstrated decreased systolic function in diabetic subjects who did not have left ventricular hypertrophy [48]. Although diastolic dysfunction is the hallmark of diabetic cardiomyopathy, concomitant subtle systolic dysfunction is present even at earlier stages of the disease.

Hyperglycemia is one of the major causes of diabetic cardiomyopathy. In the Strong Heart Study, the degree and frequency of diastolic dysfunction were directly proportional to the HbA_{1c} [49]. The most likely reason for this association is that chronic hyperglycemia leads to irreversible glycosylation of collagen, which results in increased collagen cross-linking and increased myocardial fibrosis. The presence of permanently glycosylated proteins also up-regulates receptors for advanced glycosylated end products, which also leads to myocardial fibrosis [50]. In animal studies, myocardial fibrosis decreased and diastolic function improved when collagen cross-linking was reversed with the cross-link breaker ALT-711 [51].

Intramyocellular myocardial glycation also alters calcium homeostasis, which can be reversed with aminoguanidine, which decreases the formation of permanently glycosylated proteins [52]. The myocardium of the diabetic patient in many ways resembles the ischemic myocardium in which there is decreased glucose uptake and oxidation and increased fatty acid oxygenation. Due to these changes, the ability of the myocardium to metabolize pyruvate, which is a product of glycolysis, results in a shift toward glycogen synthesis [53]. Because ATP derived from glycolysis is used for Ca^{++} uptake in the sarcoplasmic reticulum, decreases in ATP generation lead not only to decreased Ca^{++} uptake but also to rigidity of the myocardium and diastolic dysfunction [54]. In vitro studies have shown that when glycolysis is inhibited there is impaired myocardial relaxation, especially when the myocardium is ischemic or has been reperfused; inhibition of glycolysis also results in ventricular hypertrophy [53].

Hyperglycemia is also associated with an increased myocardial content of free radicals and oxidants, which results in decreased nitric oxide levels, damaged DNA, worsened endothelial function, and stimulation of poly-(ADP-ribose) polymerase-1 (PARP) [55]. Stimulation of PARP results in an up-regulation of proinflammatory pathways as well as decreased myocardial NADPH; therefore, the cellular energy pool is decreased [56].

Another interesting and recently reported effect of hyperglycemia on the myocardium is inhibition of the binding of copper to ceruloplasmin and albumin. This inhibition results in an increased intracellular copper level leading to increased free radical formation which in the myocardium causes left ventricular hypertrophy and myocardial fibrosis [57]. Evidence for this association has come from chelation experiments in humans and animals. Trietine, a selective copper chelating agent, improves cardiac structure in rats and left ventricular hypertrophy in humans [58]. Furthermore, levels of superoxide dismutase (a marker of vascular injury) and serum copper levels are correlated in the diabetic patient and are decreased with chelation therapy [58].

Mechanisms other than hyperglycemia also have a role in the development of diabetic cardiomyopathy because, in diabetic children, echocardiographically documented ventricular dysfunction does not correlate with either the HbA_{1c} level or the duration of diabetes [46]. The metabolic factor other than hyperglycemia that most likely has a role in the development of diabetic cardiomyopathy is lipotoxicity, that is, the extracellular and intracellular elevations of free fatty acids (FFAs) and triglycerides that are associated with insulin resistance and diabetes. Excess FFAs, at least in rat models, accumulate in the diabetic myocardium due to an increased extraction [53]. A breakdown product of the metabolism of FFAs, ceramide, induces the production of nitric oxide to pathologic levels, which increases the production of mitochondrial superoxide anion leading to oxidative stress [53]. Through abnormal gene expression and altered signal transduction, oxidative stress leads to activation of pathways that result in apoptosis (programmed cell death) of the cardiomyocyte [59]. Furthermore, accumulation of FFAs induces activation of the PPAR alpha receptor, which in animal models through gene overexpression has been shown to induce a cardiac dysfunction that is similar to the dysfunction seen in diabetic cardiomyopathy in humans [60,61]. Suppression of the PPAR delta may also have a role, because in animal studies PPAR delta–deficient hearts show deficient FFA oxidation and a lipotoxic cardiomyopathy that is associated with ventricular hypertrophy. These effects can be reversed with activation of the PPAR delta receptor [62].

The combination of hyperglycemia and hyperlipidemia in the diabetic patient leads to subclinical diastolic dysfunction and a subtle systolic dysfunction, both of which are worsened by an increased myocardial collagen content [38]. The subclinical myocardial dysfunction caused by diabetic cardiomyopathy is worsened by the presence of hypertension, which can potentially further damage myocardial contractile proteins, increase myocardial fibrosis, and increase hypertrophy of the ventricular myocardium [63]. Although 70% of older patients with type 2 diabetes have hypertension, even in the absence of hypertension, owing to the growth-promoting action of insulin there is a high prevalence of ventricular hypertrophy. In cross-sectional studies, 32% of new-onset type 2 diabetic non-hypertensive patients had left ventricular hypertrophy on echocardiography, and in another echocardiographic study, 71% of diabetic patients at various stages of the disease had left ventricular hypertrophy [64–67].

The addition of myocardial ischemia may change a clinically mild ventricular dysfunction due to diabetic cardiomyopathy, hypertension, and left ventricular hypertrophy into severe ventricular dysfunction, HF, and death [68]; therefore, the presence of diabetic HF requires evaluation for the presence of significant coronary artery disease.

A subset of diabetic patients with HF have little or no significant coronary artery disease, suggesting that diabetic microangiopathy may be the cause of myocardial ischemia and HF. Microvascular impairment, similar to diabetic retinopathy and nephropathy at the capillary level, has been excluded by the absence of increased lactate production during rapid atrial pacing [69]; however, it is still possible that in the diabetic patient at a more proximal site endothelial dysfunction could lead to repeated episodes of vasoconstriction leading to reperfusion injuries and eventually myocardial dysfunction [70]. Furthermore, endothelial dysfunction is also associated with increased small vessel permeability which could lead to interstitial edema, fibrosis, and myocardial dysfunction [71]. A 6-year follow-up study using retinal photography showed that the incidence of HF was significantly higher (15.1% versus 4.8%) in the diabetic patient when retinopathy was present, and that the association of retinopathy with HF persisted after adjustment for age, gender, race, the presence of coronary artery disease, hypertension, and glycemic control [72]. These studies suggest that, through endothelial dysfunction, microvascular disease has a role in the development of diabetic cardiomyopathy and HF. Another possibility is that the angiogenic response to ischemia is diminished in the diabetic patient with microangiopathy, leading to myocardial injury, fibrosis, and dysfunction [73].

Further evidence that the high prevalence (50% to 60%) of diastolic dysfunction in the type 2 diabetic patient is related to endothelial dysfunction in addition to metabolic factors can be found in the Strong Heart Study in which, in a diabetic Native American population, the only independent risk factors for the presence of diastolic dysfunction were an elevated HbA_{1c} level and the presence of microalbuminuria [49,74]. Microalbuminuria has been shown to be a marker for endothelial dysfunction. If there is endothelial dysfunction in the glomerulus and excessive albumin leaks into the renal tubule, throughout the vasculature, the endothelium is permeable to lipoproteins, monocytes, and other pro-atherogenic factors [75]. Because of this association with endothelial dysfunction, microalbuminuria has been shown to be associated with increased cardiac events and mortality [76].

The end result of the combination of diabetic cardiomyopathy, hypertension/left ventricular hypertrophy, and myocardial macrovascular and microvascular disease is a fibrotic, non-compliant myocardium that clinically first manifests as diastolic dysfunction followed by a mild but later severe systolic dysfunction. In addition, if the fibrosis extends to the papillary muscle, mitral insufficiency develops, which adds a mechanical burden to an already dysfunctional myocardium [77].

Autonomic dysfunction

In animals, experimental diabetic cardiomyopathy results in molecular and biochemical abnormalities that are similar to the changes that would occur in the myocardium due to HF caused by hemodynamic overload [78]. Pathways such as the protein kinase C and the mitogen-activated protein kinase are stimulated by mechanical stretch and by the dysmetabolism associated with hyperglycemia. The resulting changes lead to decreased myocardial performance and stimulation of the RAS and SNS, which in an acute hypotensive situation is protective and avoids hypoperfusion of vital organs. Chronic activation of the RAS and SNS and other autocrine and paracrine systems leads to accelerated apoptosis and necrosis of the cardiomyocyte. The loss of cardiomyocytes, in turn, leads to further myocardial dysfunction, further stimulation of the RAS and SNS, and a downward spiral to HF. Activation of the RAS and SNS also leads to a compensatory change in the size and shape of the ventricular chambers through cellular hypertrophy (remodeling). Despite the increased muscle mass that occurs with remodeling, the changes in cellular and extracellular composition, geometry, and energetics lead to a further decrease in ventricular function and an even greater increase in the activity of the RAS and SNS [79]. The HF that occurs with diabetic cardiomyopathy occurs in a pattern that is similar to other etiologies of HF in that an initially adaptive but later harmful process leads to progressive ventricular dysfunction.

At a cellular level, stimulation of the RAS and the SNS leads to defects in β-adrenergic receptor signal transduction which stimulates production of the mitochondrial enzyme carnitine palmityl-transferase-1 (CPT-1), which facilitates the entry of FFAs into the mitochondria. Increased use by the myocardial mitochondria of FFAs results in uncoupling of oxidative phosphorylation, inhibition of membrane ATPase activity, and increased myocardial oxygen consumption. The resulting increase in myocardial workload leads to myocardial ischemia, impaired myocardial function, and cardiac arrhythmias [80,81].

Altered gene expression

At the cellular level, activation of the RAS and SNS leads to induction of the fetal gene program, which contributes to the progression of HF. Atrial natriuretic peptide (ANP), the expression of which is confined to the atria in the healthy adult, is re-expressed in the ventricle as it was during fetal life. In the ventricle, isoforms of the fast (α) and slow (β) myosin heavy chains are changed to a fetal pattern with higher β and lower α expression. In addition, genes such as that for skeletal muscle α actin and cardiac actin, which are not expressed after birth, are re-expressed in the ventricle. The gene encoding a key ionotrophic protein, sarcoplasmic reticular Ca^{2+} ATPase (*SERCA-2*), is also down-regulated. These changes in gene expression result in a decrease in ventricular function owing to a reduction in the energy needs of the myocardium, which may initially be a an adaptive mechanism that protects the surviving myocardium but chronically leads to worsened ventricular function [82].

The altered gene expression of the fetal gene program is reversed with blockade of the RAS and SNS. Diabetic rats with beta-blockade have shown improvements in *SERCA-2* expression in addition to other aspects of fetal gene expression [83]. Because both RAS and SNS activity are increased in the diabetic and insulin resistant subject, it is likely that the altered gene expression of the fetal gene program occurs even in controlled diabetes but the addition of uncontrolled diabetes causes further stimulation. Any medication that blocks the RAS or SNS in addition to glycemic control reverses the fetal gene program and improves ventricular function.

Mitochondrial dysfunction

Mitochondrial dysfunction has a pivotal role in HF because mitochondria are the main source of reactive oxygen species, and any treatment that improves mitochondrial function can be lifesaving [84]. It can also be postulated that a major factor in the high incidence of HF in insulin resistant or diabetic patients is mitochondrial dysfunction.

Mitochondrial DNA mutations and mutations of nuclear DNA encoding for mitochondrial function have been described in maternal diabetes with deafness as well as in maturity onset diabetes of youth. Patients with these forms of diabetes and their family members demonstrate an OXPHOS defect [85]. HF is associated with increased mitochondrial DNA mutations, which may represent an accelerated ageing phenomenon because mitochondrial dysfunction increases with age. These mutations affect antioxidant gene expression and are associated with HF because mitochondrial oxidative stress accelerates cardiomyocyte apoptosis [84].

Insulin resistance has also been associated with mitochondrial dysfunction. The mitochondrial defect that has been associated with insulin resistance has been identified as affecting PPG-1, which is a co-factor for the PPAR gamma receptor [86]. PPG-1 causes decreased mitochondrial oxidative phosphorylation, facilitating the accumulation of triglyceride and related lipid molecules in muscle. The PPG-1 defect has been identified in situations in which insulin resistance is increased, such as the offspring of type 2 diabetic subjects, the elderly, and insulin resistant and type 2 diabetic subjects [87,88]. In the non-insulin resistant normoglycemic subject, voluntary muscle has a high mitochondrial content, a high lipid oxidative capacity, and little stored triglycerides, because the metabolism of triglycerides depends on transportation into the mitochondria through the activity of CPT-1. With insulin resistance, these actions are reduced, and triglyceride accumulates in the muscle, liver, and pancreatic beta cells. A breakdown product of increased cellular fatty acid metabolism, ceramide, has been shown to increase nitric oxide to intracellular levels that are toxic and accelerate apoptosis. In the diabetic patient, mitochondrial function that is already decreased with insulin resistance is further decreased due to hyperglycemia and elevated serum FFA levels [89].

Insulin resistance (metabolic syndrome)

There are many similarities between the insulin resistance syndrome and HF. Both HF and insulin resistance are increasing in prevalence, which matches the increased prevalence of obesity. In insulin resistance and HF, the RAS and SNS are activated, and both conditions are inflammatory states associated with elevated cytokines and endothelial dysfunction, obesity, hypertension, and left ventricular hypertrophy. In the Strong Heart Study, fasting insulin levels were proportional to left ventricular size and function, and regardless of whether diabetes was present, the ejection fraction was inversely proportional to insulin resistance [17,23,90,91]. A prospective study has also shown that the presence of insulin resistance is a major predictor of CHF [23].

Although there is more CHF in diabetic patients owing to hypertension/left ventricular hypertrophy, coronary artery disease, and diabetic cardiomyopathy, there is also an increased prevalence of diabetes in patients with CHF owing to activation of the RAS and SNS leading to insulin resistance [92]. A third category may be patients with defective mitochondrial function owing to a genetic predisposition that is exacerbated by aging, hyperglycemia, and elevated FFAs.

Inflammation, diabetes, and insulin resistance

Type 2 diabetes, insulin resistance, obesity, and HF are all inflammatory states that can be improved with therapies that reduce inflammation. For example, thiazolidinediones reduce highly sensitive C-reactive protein levels in diabetic and insulin resistant patients, and statins improve outcomes in CHF patients through decreasing neurohormonal activation, improving brain natriuretic peptide (BNP) levels, and increasing the left ventricular ejection fraction [93–95]. The inflammation associated with HF may be due to the accumulation in the myocardium of mast cells which accumulate after myocardial injury, especially in the atria close to capillaries.

Degranulation of these mast cells is thought to mediate reperfusion injury. Mast cell degranulation can be stabilized with anti-inflammatory medications such as antihistamines, dichromoglycate, and the highly anti-inflammatory combined alpha- and beta-blocker carvedilol [96,97].

Screening for congestive heart failure in the diabetic population

The presence of diabetes places a patient in the highest risk category for HF, and the high prevalence and significant morbidity and mortality that occurs with HF mandates its early identification so that appropriate therapy can be initiated. At least 50% of individuals with left ventricular systolic dysfunction—the antecedent to HF—are undiagnosed and more importantly untreated [98]. Diabetes has such an important influence on the development of HF that it has been incorporated as a risk factor for HF in the American College of Cardiology/American Heart Association HF guidelines [99]. In addition, the Joint National Committee on Prevention, Detection, Evaluation, and Treatment of High Blood Pressure VII report places patients with diabetes in the highest risk category for HF, even with high normal blood pressure and no target organ damage [100]. Other independent risk factors for HF in the diabetic patient are older age, longer duration of diabetes, obesity, the use of insulin, and the presence of retinopathy or albuminuria [101,102].

Screening for CHF and early ventricular function in the diabetic patient is difficult on clinical grounds. Twenty percent of diabetic subjects with an ejection fraction of under 45% have no symptoms, and in the SOLVD trial of patients with an ejection fraction under 45%, only 32% had rales, 25% had edema, 26% had neck vein distension, and 17% had an S_3 gallop [103]. Although the cardinal symptom of diastolic dysfunction is dyspnea, many diabetic HF patients lack symptoms because of inactivity. Simply walking the patient in the office or a graded exercise test can be revealing [104]. Screening of patients with a BNP level may be helpful. Like ANP, BNP is elevated with increased cardiac filling but unlike ANP is not affected by hyperglycemia [105]. When used as a screening tool in patients aged more than 55 years, BNP had a sensitivity of 92% and a specificity of 72% [106]. Plasma BNP may be an economic test that at an early stage identifies diabetic subjects with ventricular dysfunction who should be further evaluated with echocardiography.

Treatment of heart failure in the diabetic patient

Glycemic control

In the diabetic HF patient, control of hyperglycemia results in better ventricular performance through decreasing myocardial FFA use, increasing glucose use, and decreasing the cardiac workload. A recent study of fasting glucose in diabetic and non-diabetic subjects showed that the fasting glucose was an independent predictor for hospitalization for HF. In that study, for each 18 mg/dL (1 mmole) increase in fasting glucose, there was a 10% increase in the risk of hospitalization for HF [92].

The heart has a continued need for high-energy phosphates to provide energy but has a limited ability to store substrate. The heart on a daily basis generates 5 kg of ATP and completely exhausts its supply of ATP every 13 seconds [107,108]. As sources of fuel, the heart oxidizes FFAs, glucose, and lactate. Due to the high yield from the oxidation of FFAs, FFAs are preferentially used (high octane fuel). Glucose, on the other hand, is a more efficient fuel because there is a higher yield of ATP per oxygen atom in its metabolism (low octane fuel) [109]. When heart failure occurs, to reduce the cardiac workload, the heart must shift away from using FFAs and toward using glucose as a substrate for the generation of ATP, which is achieved by downregulating transcription factors for FFA metabolism [110]. In HF patients, dichloroacetate, by stimulating pyruvate dehydrogenase, the pivotal enzyme connecting glycolysis with the Kreb's cycle, decreases lactate and FFA use, increases glucose oxidation, and improves left ventricular performance [111]. Similarly, trimetazidine, by inhibiting FFA oxidation, increases the phosphocreatine to ATP ratio, indicating the preservation of myocardial high-energy phosphate levels in diabetic HF patients. As a result of this preservation, trimetazidine improves the ejection fraction, the New York Heart Association (NYHA) functional class, diastolic dysfunction, quality of life, angina frequency, and endothelial function, and decreases systolic and diastolic cardiac diameters [112].

The high FFA levels that accompany hyperglycemia in the diabetic patient also have the potential to be cardiotoxic through disrupting plasma membrane structure and function and increasing intracellular calcium and the cardiac workload [113,114]. Elevated FFAs also increase cardiac sympathetic activity and the risk of arrhythmia [115].

The action of insulin itself rather than its ability to lower glucose and FFA levels may have a pivotal role in ventricular function. Insulin through binding to its receptor on the myocardium activates a cascade of chemical changes that result in the generation of protein kinase B (also called Akt-1), which stimulates nitric oxide production and myocardial hypertrophy and inhibits apoptosis. When insulin resistance is present, there is less nitric oxide production, increased apoptosis, and less myocyte formation [116].

The lowering of glucose and FFA levels and the action of insulin itself should result in improved myocardial function in the diabetic HF patient. Although the potential of glycemic control to improve ventricular function has never been fully studied, based on pathophysiologic and epidemiologic evidence and clinical observation, aggressive glycemic control should be part of the comprehensive management strategy in any diabetic HF patient.

Use of thiazolidinediones, biguanides, and incretin mimetics

Thiazolidinediones increase fluid retention, especially at higher doses and when used in combination with medications such as insulin or sulfonylureas which increase serum insulin levels. Thiazolidinediones increase fluid and sodium retention through their effect on the distal renal tubule. Owing to this site of action, loop and thiazide diuretics are ineffective in reducing fluid retention, whereas spironolactone can be effective [117]. Because insulin also acts at a different site of the renal tubule to retain sodium, the effects of insulin itself or high insulin levels induced by the secretagogues are additive to those of the thiazolidinediones [117]. The retention of fluid usually results in dependent edema that is easily distinguished from HF by clinical examination or by obtaining a serum BNP level. Nevertheless, thiazolidinedione-induced fluid retention can result in as much as a 6% increase in plasma volume, and in a diabetic subject with diastolic dysfunction, the increased filling pressure can precipitate HF. The incidence of HF in studies of thiazolidinediones is less than 1%, and, indeed, the increase in plasma volume that results from fluid retention might be regarded as a "stress test" for the stiffened myocardium. With thiazolidinedione use, HF might be diagnosed and treated several months or years before the HF would become clinically obvious. Thiazolidinediones have no adverse effect on the myocardium itself and have been shown to preserve or even marginally improve the ejection fraction and do not cause left ventricular hypertrophy, at least in NYHA class 1 and 2 subjects [118].

Because no studies have been preformed in NYHA class 3 and 4 subjects with HF, thiazolidinediones are contraindicated with these classifications. Nevertheless, thiazolidinediones may improve the outcomes in patients with advanced HF. In a Medicare billing study, when thiazolidinediones were used in hospitalized patients with CHF (of whom more than 70% had pulmonary edema, a group for whom thiazolidinediones are definitely contraindicated), there was a 13% decrease in mortality but a 6% increase in the rate of readmission with HF [119].

Due to the perceived risk of lactic acidosis, the use of metformin is contraindicated in HF. Nevertheless, data also derived from Medicare billing have shown that hospitalized HF patients discharged on metformin had a 13% decrease in mortality and, if thiazolidinedione was used with metformin, a 24% decrease in mortality. Readmissions with metformin monotherapy were nonsignificantly reduced by 8% [119]. Confirmation of these surprising findings has been obtained from prescription data in Saskatchewan, Canada. Diabetic HF patients who used metformin had at 1 year a decreased mortality (14% versus 26%) and at 2.5 years a 30% reduction in mortality when compared with patients using sulfonylureas [120]. In the Kaiser Permanente Northwest Diabetes Registry, the incidence of the development of CHF was lowest with metformin when compared with the use of insulin or sulfonylureas [121].

The reason for the improved outcome for diabetic HF patients on metformin or a thiazolidinedione is thought to be due to increased intracellular levels of 5-AMP-activated protein kinase (5-AMPK). 5-AMPK can be regarded as a "fuel gauge" enzyme that is activated by energy consumption. When intracellular ATP levels are low, activation of 5-AMPK will result in an increased cellular ATP level due to increased production and decreased breakdown of ATP. In skeletal muscle, 5-AMPK is activated with exercise and is involved in contraction-stimulated glucose transport and FFA oxidation. During myocardial ischemia, 5-AMPK activity increases, which in the myocardium sustains viability and function. In the liver, 5-AMPK inhibits glucose, cholesterol, and triglyceride synthesis and stimulates FFA oxidation. In rodents, 5-AMPK activation lowers glucose, cholesterol, and blood pressure levels. Metformin stimulates 5-AMPK activity directly, whereas thiazolidinediones probably stimulate 5-AMPK activity through increased adiponectin levels, which, in turn, is due to a thiazolidinedione-stimulated increase in production from peritoneal adipocytes [122].

Obviously, further prospective research into the use of metformin or thiazolidinediones with HF is needed before their use in the diabetic HF patient can be recommended or even considered. Drugs such as thiazolidinediones and metformin may also through lowering of insulin resistance improve the outcome for the diabetic HF patient. Exercise, the best nonpharmacologic method of lowering insulin resistance, has clearly been shown in a meta-analysis of HF patients to reduce mortality and the rate of hospital readmissions [123]. Similarly, weight loss results in an improvement in diastolic and systolic ventricular function [124]. Lowering of insulin resistance may facilitate the insulin-induced entry of glucose into the myocardiocyte, shifting the metabolism of the myocardium away from the use of FFA and toward the use of glucose and resulting in a decrease in the cardiac workload, an improvement in ventricular function, and an increase in survival [125].

A new class of anti-diabetic drugs, the incretin mimetics, may also be of benefit in HF. Incretins are secreted from specialized gut endocrine cells and increase glucose-dependent insulin secretion. The most important incretin is glucagon-like peptide (GLP-1), which is rapidly metabolized by the enzyme dipeptyl peptidase 4 (DPP4). Exenatide given by injection is resistant to the action of DPP4 and mimics the effect of GLP-1, whereas sitagliptin is an oral preparation that, by inhibiting DPP4 activity, raises GLP-1 levels.

The effects of GLP-1 are not restricted to the pancreas and the gastrointestinal tract. In animal studies and in HF patients, GLP-1 when given intravenously through its cardiac receptors has been shown to improve the ejection fraction and regional wall scores, dilate the pulmonary artery, and have a diuretic effect [126,127].

Agents used to treat heart failure in the diabetic patient

Diuretics and digoxin improve the clinical manifestations of HF and improve the quality of life for the HF patient; however, their use does not improve mortality. To improve mortality in the diabetic HF patient, ventricular remodeling must at least be halted and preferably reversed. It is therefore imperative that drugs that suppress the RAS and SNS be used, especially in the diabetic patient in whom these systems are overactivated. With reversal of remodeling, there will be improvements in mortality and morbidity in the diabetic HF patient.

Angiotensin-converting enzyme inhibitors

Angiotensin II through its type 1 receptor in addition to being a potent vasoconstrictor causes cardiomyocyte hypertrophy and the formation of collagen by cardiac fibroblasts, leading to myocardial fibrosis [128]. The angiotensin II type 1 receptor is also stimulated by high insulin levels in the diabetic and insulin resistant patient [129]. ACE inhibitors prevent the formation of angiotensin II and attenuate myocardial hypertrophy and fibrosis by elevating bradykinin and prostacycline levels and releasing nitric oxide [130]. Although ACE inhibitors prevent myocardial remodeling, the remodeling is not reversed [131].

ACE inhibitors are at least as effective in reducing mortality in the diabetic HF patient as in the non-diabetic HF patient. High-dose lisinopril in the ATLAS trial resulted in a 51% lowering of morality in diabetic HF patients [27]. In the SAVE study, captopril lowered mortality as much in diabetic patients as non-diabetic HF patients, and in the GISSI-3 study, lisinopril resulted in a significantly greater lowering of mortality in diabetic HF patients when compared with their non-diabetic peers [132,133]. In the TRACE study, trandolapril significantly lowered the event rate by 62% in diabetic HF patients, whereas it did not significantly lower the event rate in non-diabetic HF patients (the risk was lowered by only 19%) [134]. These studies suggest that ACE inhibitors are at least as powerful in decreasing mortality and cardiac events in the diabetic HF patient as in the non-diabetic HF patient.

Angiotensin receptor blockers

The use of angiotensin receptor blockers in HF associated with diabetes has produced mixed results. Losartan use in the RENAAL (Reduction of Endpoints in NIDDM with Angiotensin II Antagonist Losartan) trial resulted in the rate for first hospitalization with HF being significantly reduced by 32% without a significant effect on cardiovascular events or mortality [135]. On the other hand, the CHARM (Candesartan in Heart Failure Assessment of Reduction in Mortality and Morbidity) trial showed that with systolic dysfunction, candesartan used without an ACE inhibitor decreased cardiovascular mortality and hospitalizations for HF by 23%. When added to an ACE inhibitor, cardiovascular death and hospitalizations were significantly reduced by 15% [136]. In addition, when candesartan was used in diastolic dysfunction, HF hospitalizations were significantly reduced [137]. Although specific information on the outcomes in diabetic HF patients included in this study is not available, the rate of new-onset diabetes was reduced, more than offsetting the increase in new-onset diabetes that is to be expected with HF [138,139].

Overall, in the diabetic HF patient, the use of an ACE inhibitor is preferred over an angiotensin receptor blocker; however, an angiotensin receptor blocker can be substituted for an ACE inhibitor when intolerable side effects of an ACE inhibitor occur, and an angiotensin receptor blocker can also be safely added to an ACE inhibitor to further suppress the RAS in the HF patient. The fear that mortality can increase when an angiotensin receptor blocker is added to the combination of an ACE inhibitor and a beta-blocker, found on a retrospective analysis of the use of valsartan in the VALHEF trial, is irrational based on the results of the prospective CHARM Added trial in which candesartan was added to an ACE inhibitor [137,138].

Aldosterone antagonists

Aldosterone is produced in excess in HF in an attempt to correct renal hypoperfusion; however, excess aldosterone results in inflammation, hypertrophic fibrosis, ischemia of the myocardium, and ventricular arrhythmias [140]. Both the nonspecific aldosterone antagonist spironolactone and the selective aldosterone antagonist eplerenone have been shown to improve mortality in patients with advanced HF and may benefit patients with mild HF [141,142]. The downside of aldosterone antagonists is that the potential for life-threatening hyperkalemia increases dramatically. When the use of spironolactone was shown to benefit HF, admissions to the hospital for hyperkalemia increased [143]. Hyperkalemia is most likely to occur with renal insufficiency and severe HF but may also occur in the diabetic patient with normal renal function owing to an increased prevalence of type 4 renal tubular acidosis (hyporeninemic hypoaldosteronism) in these subjects [144]. If an aldosterone antagonist is used in a diabetic patient, monitoring of the serum potassium should be preformed at days 3, 10, and 21 after initiation.

Beta-blockers

Blockade of the SNS not only prevents but also reverses myocardial remodeling; however, unlike blockade of the RAS in the diabetic HF patient, in whom events and mortality may be reduced even further, the use of beta-blockers in the diabetic HF patient does not seem to be as effective as it is in the non-diabetic HF patient [145]. A meta-analysis of the effects of beta-blockers on all-cause mortality showed a significant 28% risk reduction in the non-diabetic HF subject and a significant 16% risk reduction in the diabetic HF subject, with the difference between the diabetic and non-diabetic HF subjects being statistically significant [145].

On further inspection of the data, in the trials in which the combined alpha- and beta-blocker carvedilol was used, there was the same reduced mortality in the diabetic HF patient as there was in the non-diabetic HF patient. A meta-analysis of placebo-controlled HF trials with carvedilol showed that there was no significant difference in mortality between diabetic and non-diabetic HF subjects [35]. In the meta-analysis, the number of patients that needed to be treated for 1 year to avoid one death was 23 in the non-diabetic HF group and 25 in the diabetic HF group. These differences might be accounted for by total beta- rather than just β_1-blockade, the addition of α_1-blockade, or the anti-inflammatory and antioxidant effects of carvedilol. Carvedilol also has the advantage of improving insulin resistance and not worsening glycemic control in the diabetic patient; therefore, it should be the beta-blocker of choice in the diabetic HF patient [146].

Summary

Diabetic patients have a higher incidence and prevalence of HF as well as a worse prognosis from HF when compared with non-diabetic HF patients. The cardiotoxic triad of diabetic cardiomyopathy, hypertension/ventricular hypertrophy, and more severe and extensive coronary artery disease that occurs in the diabetic patient leads to the increased frequency of and worsened prognosis from HF. Glycemic control may improve cardiac metabolism and myocardial function in the diabetic HF patient. Blockade of the RAS and the SNS at the earliest possible stage is essential to prevent and reverse myocardial remodeling. The improvement in cardiac function that results from blockade of these systems will result in decreases in morbidity and mortality in the diabetic patient with HF that are at least as great as those in the non-diabetic HF patient. Earlier diagnosis and more aggressive therapy to improve ventricular dysfunction will result in an improved outcome for the diabetic patient with HF.

References

[1] Bell DS. Drugs for cardiovascular risk reduction in the diabetic patient. Curr Diab Rep 2001;1(2):133–9.
[2] Expert Panel on Detection, Evaluation, and Treatment of High Blood Cholesterol in Adults. Executive summary of the third report of the National Cholesterol Education Program (NCEP) Expert Panel On Detection, Evaluation, and Treatment of High Blood Cholesterol in Adults (Adult Treatment Panel III). JAMA 2001;285(19):2486–97.
[3] Haffner SM, Lehto S, Rönnemaa T, et al. Mortality from coronary heart disease in subjects with type 2 diabetes and in nondiabetic subjects with and without prior myocardial infarction. N Engl J Med 1998;339(4):229–34.
[4] Miettinen H, Lehto S, Salomaa V, et al. Impact of diabetes on mortality after the first myocardial infarction: the FINMONICA Myocardial Infarction Register Study Group. Diabetes Care 1998;21(1):69–75.
[5] Lewis EF, Moye LA, Rouleau JL, et al. CARE Study. Predictors of late development of heart failure in stable survivors of myocardial infarction: the CARE study. J Am Coll Cardiol 2003;42(8):1446–53.
[6] Kannel WB, McGee DL. Diabetes and cardiovascular disease: the Framingham study. JAMA 1979;241(19):2035–8.
[7] Cook CB, Tsui C, Ziemer DC, et al. Common reasons for hospitalization among adult patients with diabetes. Endocr Pract 2006;12(4):363–70.
[8] Reis SE, Holubkov R, Edmundowicz D, et al. Treatment of patients admitted to the hospital with congestive heart failure: specialty-related disparities in practice patterns and outcomes. J Am Coll Cardiol 1997;30(3):733–8.
[9] Kannel WB, Hjortland M, Castelli WP. Role of diabetes in congestive heart failure: the Framingham study. Am J Cardiol 1974;34(1):29–34.

[10] Zarich SW, Nesto RW. Diabetic cardiomyopathy. Am Heart J 1989;118(5 Pt 1):1000–12.

[11] Nichols GA, Hillier TA, Erbey JR, et al. Congestive heart failure in type 2 diabetes: prevalence, incidence, and risk factors. Diabetes Care 2001;24(9): 1614–9.

[12] Aronow WS, Ahn C. Incidence of heart failure in 2737 older persons with and without diabetes mellitus. Chest 1999;115(3):867–8.

[13] Amato L, Paolisso G, Cacciatore F, et al. Congestive heart failure predicts the development of non-insulin-dependent diabetes mellitus in the elderly: the Observatorio Geriatrico Regione Campania Group. Diabetes Metab 1997;23(3):213–8.

[14] Stratton IM, Adler AI, Neil HA, et al. Association of glycaemia with macrovascular and microvascular complications of type 2 diabetes (UKPDS 35): prospective observational study. BMJ 2000; 321(7258):405–12.

[15] Adams KF Jr, Fonarow GC, Emerman CL, et al. ADHERE Scientific Advisory Committee and Investigators. Characteristics and outcomes of patients hospitalized for heart failure in the United States: rationale, design, and preliminary observations from the first 100,000 cases in the Acute Decompensated Heart Failure National Registry (ADHERE). Am Heart J 2005;149(2):209–16.

[16] Bell DSH, Ovalle F. Frequency of diabetes in patients admitted to hospital because of congestive heart failure [abstract]. Diabetes 2001;50:A456.

[17] Bertoni AG, Tsai A, Kasper EK, et al. Diabetes and idiopathic cardiomyopathy: a nationwide case-control study. Diabetes Care 2003;26(10): 2791–5.

[18] Suskin N, McKelvie RS, Burns RJ, et al. Glucose and insulin abnormalities relate to functional capacity in patients with congestive heart failure. Eur Heart J 2000;21(16):1368–75.

[19] Kemppainen J, Tsuchida H, Stolen K, et al. Insulin signaling and resistance in patients with chronic heart failure. J Physiol 2003;550(Pt1):305–15.

[20] Witteles RM, Tang WH, Jamali AH, et al. Insulin resistance in idiopathic dilated cardiomyopathy: a possible etiologic link. J Am Coll Cardiol 2004; 44(1):78–81.

[21] Swan JN, Ankers D, Walton C, et al. Insulin resistance in chronic heart failure: relation to severity and etiology of heart failure. J Am Coll Cardiol 1997;30(2):527–32.

[22] Arnlöv J, Lind L, Zethelius B, et al. Several factors associated with the insulin resistance syndrome are predictors of left ventricular systolic dysfunction in a male population after 20 years of follow-up. Am Heart J 2001;142(4):720–4.

[23] Ingelsson E, Sundström J, Arnlöv J, et al. Insulin resistance and risk of congestive heart failure. JAMA 2005;294(3):334–41.

[24] The CONSENSUS Trial Study Group. Effects of enalapril on mortality in severe congestive heart failure: results of the Cooperative North Scandinavian Enalapril Survival Study. N Engl J Med 1987; 316(23):1429–35.

[25] The SOLVD Investigators. Effect of enalapril on survival in patients with reduced left ventricular ejection fractions and congestive heart failure. N Engl J Med 1991;325(5):293–302.

[26] Cohn JN, Johnson G, Ziesche S, et al. A comparison of enalapril with hydralazine-isosorbide dinitrate in the treatment of chronic congestive heart failure. N Engl J Med 1991;325(5): 303–10.

[27] Packer M, Poole-Wilson PA, Armstrong PW, et al. Comparative effects of low and high doses of the angiotensin-converting enzyme inhibitor, lisinopril, on morbidity and mortality in chronic heart failure: ATLAS Study Group. Circulation 1999; 100(23):2312–8.

[28] The Cardiac Insufficiency Bisoprolol Study II (CIBIS-II): a randomised trial. Lancet 1999; 353(9146):9–13.

[29] Domanski M, Krause-Steinrauf H, Deedwania P, et al. BEST Investigators. The effect of diabetes on outcomes of patients with advanced heart failure in the BEST trial. J Am Coll Cardiol 2003; 42(5):914–22.

[30] Effect of metoprolol CR/XL in chronic heart failure: Metoprolol CR/XL Randomised Intervention Trial in Congestive Heart Failure (MERIT-HF). Lancet 1999;353(9169):2001–7.

[31] Randomised, placebo-controlled trial of carvedilol in patients with congestive heart failure due to ischaemic heart disease: Australia/New Zealand Heart Failure Research Collaborative Group. Lancet 1997;349(9049):375–80.

[32] Colucci WS, Packer M, Bristow MR, et al. Carvedilol inhibits clinical progression in patients with mild symptoms of heart failure: US Carvedilol Heart Failure Study Group. Circulation 1996; 94(11):2800–6.

[33] Krum H, Roecker EB, Mohacsi P, et al. Carvedilol Prospective Randomized Cumulative Survival (COPERNICUS) Study Group. Effects of initiating carvedilol in patients with severe chronic heart failure: results from the COPERNICUS Study. JAMA 2003;289(6):712–8.

[34] Malmberg K, Rydén L, Efendic S, et al. Randomized trial of insulin-glucose infusion followed by subcutaneous insulin treatment in diabetic patients with acute myocardial infarction (DIGAMI study): effects on mortality at 1 year. J Am Coll Cardiol 1995;26(1):57–65.

[35] Bell DS, Lukas MA, Holdbrook FK, et al. The effect of carvedilol on mortality risk in heart failure patients with diabetes: results of a meta-analysis. Curr Med Res Opin 2006;22(2):287–96.

[36] Dries DL, Sweitzer NK, Drazner MH, et al. Prognostic impact of diabetes mellitus in patients with heart failure according to the etiology of left

ventricular systolic dysfunction. J Am Coll Cardiol 2001;38(2):421–8.

[37] Paolisso G, Tagliamonte MR, Rizzo MR, et al. Prognostic importance of insulin-mediated glucose uptake in aged patients with congestive heart failure secondary to mitral and/or aortic valve disease. Am J Cardiol 1999;83(9):1338–44.

[38] Bell DS. Heart failure: the frequent, forgotten, and often fatal complication of diabetes. Diabetes Care 2003;26(8):2433–41.

[39] Factor SM, Minase T, Sonnenblick EH. Clinical and morphological features of human hypertensive-diabetic cardiomyopathy. Am Heart J 1980; 99(4):446–58.

[40] Huggett RJ, Scott EM, Gilbey SG, et al. Impact of type 2 diabetes mellitus on sympathetic neural mechanisms in hypertension. Circulation 2003; 108(25):3097–101.

[41] Hoffman RP, Sinkey CA, Kienzle MG, et al. Muscle sympathetic nerve activity is reduced in IDDM before overt autonomic neuropathy. Diabetes 1993;42(3):375–80.

[42] Ganguly PK, Pierce GN, Dhalla KS, et al. Defective sarcoplasmic reticular calcium transport in diabetic cardiomyopathy. Am J Physiol 1983; 244(6):E528–35.

[43] Giacomelli F, Wiener J. Primary myocardial disease in the diabetic mouse: an ultrastructural study. Lab Invest 1979;40(4):460–73.

[44] Poirier P, Bogaty P, Garneau C, et al. Diastolic dysfunction in normotensive men with well-controlled type 2 diabetes: importance of maneuvers in echocardiographic screening for preclinical diabetic cardiomyopathy. Diabetes Care 2001;24(1):5–10.

[45] Sohn DW, Chai IH, Lee DJ, et al. Assessment of mitral annulus velocity by Doppler tissue imaging in the evaluation of left ventricular diastolic dysfunction. J Am Coll Cardiol 1997;30:595–602.

[46] Suys BE, Katier N, Rooman RP, et al. Female children and adolescents with type 1 diabetes have more pronounced early echocardiographic signs of diabetic cardiomyopathy. Diabetes Care 2004; 27(8):1947–53.

[47] Redfield MM, Jacobsen SJ, Burnett JC Jr, et al. Burden of systolic and diastolic ventricular dysfunction in the community: appreciating the scope of the heart failure epidemic. JAMA 2003;289(2): 194–202.

[48] Fang ZY, Yuda S, Anderson V, et al. Echocardiographic detection of early diabetic myocardial disease. J Am Coll Cardiol 2003;41(4):611–7.

[49] Devereux RB, Roman MJ, Paranicas M, et al. Impact of diabetes on cardiac structure and function: the strong heart study. Circulation 2000;101(19): 2271–6.

[50] Cooper ME. Importance of advanced glycation end products in diabetes-associated cardiovascular and renal disease. Am J Hypertens 2004;17(12 Pt 2): 31S–8S.

[51] Candido R, Forbes JM, Thomas MC, et al. A breaker of advanced glycation end products attenuates diabetes-induced myocardial structural changes. Circ Res 2003;92(7):785–92.

[52] Ziegelhoffer A, Ravingerova T, Styk J, et al. Mechanisms that may be involved in calcium tolerance of the diabetic heart. Mol Cell Biochem 1997;176(1–2): 191–8.

[53] Ungar I, Gilbert M, Siegel A, et al. Studies on myocardial metabolism. IV. Myocardial metabolism in diabetes. Am J Med 1955;18(3):385–96.

[54] Ligeti L, Szenczi O, Prestia CM, et al. Altered calcium handling is an early sign of streptozotocin-induced diabetic cardiomyopathy. Int J Mol Med 2006;17(6):1035–43.

[55] Garcia Soriano F, Virág L, Jagtap P, et al. Diabetic endothelial dysfunction: the role of poly(ADP-ribose) polymerase activation. Nat Med 2001; 7(1):108–13.

[56] Szabó C. Roles of poly(ADP-ribose) polymerase activation in the pathogenesis of diabetes mellitus and its complications. Pharmacol Res 2005;52(1): 60–71.

[57] Cooper GJ, Chan YK, Dissanayake AM, et al. Demonstration of a hyperglycemia-driven pathogenic abnormality of copper homeostasis in diabetes and its reversibility by selective chelation: quantitative comparisons between the biology of copper and eight other nutritionally essential elements in normal and diabetic individuals. Diabetes 2005;54(5):1468–76.

[58] Cooper GJ, Phillips AR, Choong SY, et al. Regeneration of the heart in diabetes by selective copper chelation. Diabetes 2004;53(9):2501–8.

[59] Singal PK, Bello-Klein A, Farahmand F, et al. Oxidative stress and functional deficit in diabetic cardiomyopathy. Adv Exp Med Biol 2001;498:213–20.

[60] Young ME, Laws FA, Goodwin GW, et al. Reactivation of peroxisome proliferator-activated receptor alpha is associated with contractile dysfunction in hypertrophied rat heart. J Biolumin Chemilumin 2001;276(48):44390–5.

[61] Finck BN, Lehman JJ, Leone TC, et al. The cardiac phenotype induced by PPAR alpha overexpression mimics that caused by diabetes mellitus. J Clin Invest 2002;109(1):121–30.

[62] Barish GD, Narkar VA, Evans RM. PPAR delta: a dagger in the heart of the metabolic syndrome. J Clin Invest 2006;116:590–7.

[63] Regan TJ, Wu CF, Yeh CK, et al. Myocardial composition and function in diabetes: the effects of chronic insulin use. Circ Res 1981;49(6):1268–77.

[64] Harris MI. Epidemiology of diabetes mellitus among the elderly in the United States. Clin Geriatr Med 1990;6(4):703–19.

[65] Struthers AD, Morris AD. Screening for and treating left-ventricular abnormalities in diabetes mellitus: a new way of reducing cardiac deaths. Lancet 2002;359(9315):1430–2.

[66] Dawson A, Morris AD, Struthers AD. The epidemiology of left ventricular hypertrophy in type 2 diabetes mellitus. Diabetologia 2005;48(10):1971–9.

[67] Sowers JR, Epstein M, Frohlich ED. Diabetes, hypertension, and cardiovascular disease: an update. Hypertension 2001;37(4):1053–9.

[68] Dash H, Johnson RA, Dinsmore RE, et al. Cardiomyopathic syndrome due to coronary artery disease. II. Increased prevalence in patients with diabetes mellitus: a matched pair analysis. Br Heart J 1977;39(7):740–7.

[69] Genda A, Mizuno S, Nunoda S, et al. Clinical studies on diabetic myocardial disease using exercise testing with myocardial scintigraphy and endomyocardial biopsy. Clin Cardiol 1986;9(8):375–82.

[70] Ahmed SS, Jaferi GA, Narang RM, et al. Preclinical abnormality of left ventricular function in diabetes mellitus. Am Heart J 1975;89(2):153–8.

[71] Factor SM. Microangiopathy and local myocardial injury: their role in the development of diabetic cardiomyopathy. In: Nagano M, Dhalla NS, editors. The diabetic heart. New York: Raven Press; 1991. p. 89–101.

[72] Wong TY, Rosamond W, Chang PP, et al. Retinopathy and risk of congestive heart failure. JAMA 2005;293(1):63–9.

[73] Yarom R, Zirkin H, Stämmler G, et al. Human coronary microvessels in diabetes and ischaemia: morphometric study of autopsy material. J Pathol 1992;166(3):265–70.

[74] Shehadeh A, Regan TJ. Cardiac consequences of diabetes mellitus. Clin Cardiol 1995;18(6):301–5.

[75] Jensen JS, Feldt-Rasmussen B, Borch-Johnsen K, et al. Increased transvascular lipoprotein transport in diabetes: association with albuminuria and systolic hypertension. J Clin Endocrinol Metab 2005; 90(8):4441–5.

[76] Yudkin JS, Forrest RD, Jackson CA. Microalbuminuria as a predictor of vascular disease in non-diabetic subjects: Islington Diabetes Survey. Lancet 1998;2(8610):530–3.

[77] Stone PH, Muller JE, Hartwell T, et al. The effect of diabetes mellitus on prognosis and serial left ventricular function after acute myocardial infarction: contribution of both coronary disease and diastolic left ventricular dysfunction to the adverse prognosis. The MILIS Study Group. J Am Coll Cardiol 1989;14(1):49–57.

[78] Bristo MR. Why does the myocardium fail? Lancet 1998;352(suppl 1):S18–24.

[79] Eichhorn EJ, Bristow MR. Medical therapy can improve the biological properties of the chronically failing heart: a new era in the treatment of heart failure. Circulation 1996;94(9):2285–96.

[80] Lopaschuk G. Regulation of carbohydrate metabolism in ischemia and reperfusion. Am Heart J 2000;139(2 Pt 3):S115–9.

[81] Panchal AR, Stanley WC, Kerner J, et al. Beta-receptor blockade decreases carnitine palmitoyl transferase I activity in dogs with heart failure. J Card Fail 1998;4(2):121–6.

[82] Bristow M. Etomoxir: a new approach to treatment of chronic heart failure. Lancet 2000;356(9242): 1621–2.

[83] Lowes BD, Gilbert EM, Abraham WT, et al. Myocardial gene expression in dilated cardiomyopathy treated with beta-blocking agents. N Engl J Med 2002;346(18):1357–65.

[84] Sheeran FL, Pepe S. Energy deficiency in the failing heart: linking increased reactive oxygen species and disruption of oxidative phosphorylation rate. Biochim Biophys Acta 2006;1757:543–52.

[85] Wallace DC. A mitochondrial paradigm of metabolic and degenerative diseases, aging, and cancer: a dawn for evolutionary medicine. Annu Rev Genet 2005;39:359–407.

[86] Peterson KF, Defour S, BeFroy D, et al. Impaired mitochondrial activity in insulin-resistant offspring of patients with type 2 diabetes. N Engl J Med 2004; 350(7):664–71.

[87] Kelley DE, He J, Menshikova EV, et al. Dysfunction of mitochondria in human skeletal muscle in type 2 diabetes. Diabetes 2002;51(10):2944–50.

[88] Petersen KF, Befroy D, Dufour S, et al. Mitochondrial dysfunction in the elderly: possible role in insulin resistance. Science 2003;300(5622):1140–2.

[89] Bell DSH. Management of type 2 diabetes with thiazolidinediones: link between B-cell preservation and durability of response. Endocrinologist 2004;4(5):293–9.

[90] Ilercil A, Devereux RB, Roman MJ, et al. Associations of insulin levels with left ventricular structure and function in American Indians: the Strong Heart Study. Diabetes 2002;51(5):1543–7.

[91] Iozzo P, Chareonthaitawee P, Dutka D, et al. Independent association of type 2 diabetes and coronary artery disease with myocardial insulin resistance. Diabetes 2002;51(10):3020–4.

[92] Held C, Gerstein HC, Yusuf S, et al. ONTARGET/ TRANSCEND Investigators. Glucose levels predict hospitalization for congestive heart failure in patients at high cardiovascular risk. Circulation 2007;115(11):1371–5.

[93] Buckingham RE. Thiazolidinediones: pleiotropic drugs with potent anti-inflammatory properties for tissue protection. Hepatol Res 2005;33(2): 167–70.

[94] Laufs U, Custodis F, Böhm M. HMG-CoA reductase inhibitors in chronic heart failure: potential mechanisms of benefit and risk. Drugs 2006;66(2): 145–54.

[95] Yamada T, Node K, Mine T, et al. Long-term effect of atorvastatin on neurohormonal activation and cardiac function in patients with chronic heart failure: a prospective randomized controlled study. Am Heart J 2007;153(6):1055e1–8.

[96] Frangogiannis NG, Lindsey ML, Michael LH, et al. Resident cardiac mast cells degranulate and

release preformed TNF-alpha, initiating the cytokine cascade in experimental canine myocardial
ischemia/reperfusion. Circulation 1998;98(7):
699–710.

[97] Keller AM, Clancy RM, Barr ML, et al. Acute
reoxygenation injury in the isolated rat heart: role
of resident cardiac mast cells. Circ Res 1988;63(6):
1044–52.

[98] McDonagh TA, Morrison CE, Lawrence A, et al.
Symptomatic and asymptomatic left ventricular
systolic dysfunction in an urban population. Lancet 1997;350(9094):829–33.

[99] Hunt SA, Baker DW, Chin MH, et al. American
College of Cardiology/American Heart Association. ACC/AHA guidelines for the evaluation and
management of chronic heart failure in the adult:
executive summary. A report of the American College of Cardiology/American Heart Association
Task Force on Practice Guidelines (Committee to
revise the 1995 Guidelines for the Evaluation and
Management of Heart Failure). J Am Coll Cardiol
2001;38(7):2101–13.

[100] Chobanian AV, Bakris GL, Black HR, et al.
National Heart, Lung, and Blood Institute Joint
National Committee on Prevention, Detection,
Evaluation, and Treatment of High Blood Pres-
sure; National High Blood Pressure Education Pro-
gram Coordinating Committee. The Seventh
Report of the Joint National Committee on Pre-
vention, Detection, Evaluation, and Treatment of
High Blood Pressure: the JNC 7 report. JAMA
2003;289(19):2560–72.

[101] Iribarren C, Karter AJ, Go AS, et al. Glycemic control and heart failure among adult patients with
diabetes. Circulation 2001;103(22):2668–73.

[102] Adler AI, Stratton IM, Neil HA, et al. Association
of systolic blood pressure with macrovascular and
microvascular complications of type 2 diabetes
(UKPDS 36): prospective observational study.
BMJ 2000;321(7258):412–9.

[103] Bourassa MG, Gurne O, Bangdiwala SI, et al. Natural history and patterns of current practice in
heart failure: the Studies of Left Ventricular Dysfunction (SOLVD) Investigators. J Am Coll Cardiol 1993;22(4 Suppl A):14A–9A.

[104] Bittner V, Weiner DH, Yusuf S, et al. Prediction of
mortality and morbidity with a 6-minute walk test
in patients with left ventricular dysfunction: SOLVD
Investigators. JAMA 1993;270(14):1702–7.

[105] McKenna K, Smith D, Tormey W, et al. Acute
hyperglycaemia causes elevation in plasma atrial
natriuretic peptide concentrations in type 1 diabetes mellitus. Diabet Med 2000;17(7):512–7.

[106] McDonagh TA, Robb SD, Murdoch DR, et al.
Biochemical detection of left-ventricular systolic
dysfunction. Lancet 1998;351(9095):9–13.

[107] Shah A, Shannon RP. Insulin resistance in dilated
cardiomyopathy. Rev Cardiovasc Med 2003;
4(Suppl 6):S50–7.

[108] Taegtmeyer H. Switching metabolic genes to
build a better heart. Circulation 2002;106(16):
2043–5.

[109] Dávila-Román VG, Vedala G, Herrero P, et al. Altered myocardial fatty acid and glucose metabolism
in idiopathic dilated cardiomyopathy. J Am Coll
Cardiol 2002;40(2):271–7.

[110] Taegtmeyer H, Hems R, Krebs HA. Utilization of
energy-providing substrates in the isolated working
rat heart. Biochem J 1980;186(3):701–11.

[111] Bersin RM, Wolfe C, Kwasman M, et al. Improved hemodynamic function and mechanical
efficiency in congestive heart failure with sodium
dichloroacetate. J Am Coll Cardiol 1994;23(7):
1617–24.

[112] Fragasso G, Perseghin G, De Cobelli F, et al.
Effects of metabolic modulation by trimetazidine
on left ventricular function and phosphocreatine/
adenosine triphosphate ratio in patients with heart
failure. Eur Heart J 2006;27(8):942–8.

[113] Oliver MF, Opie LH. Effects of glucose and fatty
acids on myocardial ischaemia and arrhythmias.
Lancet 1994;343(8890):155–8.

[114] Mjos OD. Effect of free fatty acids on myocardial
function and oxygen consumption in intact dogs.
J Clin Invest 1971;50(7):1386–9.

[115] Paolisso G, Manzella D, Rizzo MR, et al. Elevated
plasma fatty acid concentrations stimulate the cardiac autonomic nervous system in healthy subjects.
Am J Clin Nutr 2000;72(3):723–30.

[116] Lawlor MA, Alessi DR. PKB/Akt: a key mediator
of cell proliferation, survival and insulin responses?
J Cell Sci 2001;114(Pt 16):2903–10.

[117] Karalliedde J, Buckingham R, Starkie M, et al.
Rosiglitazone Fluid Retention Study Group: effect
of various diuretic treatments on rosiglitazone-
induced fluid retention. J Am Soc Nephrol 2006;
17(12):3482–90.

[118] Dargie HJ, Hildebrandt PR, Riegger GA, et al. A
randomized, placebo-controlled trial assessing the
effects of rosiglitazone on echocardiographic function and cardiac status in type 2 diabetic patients
with New York Heart Association functional class
I or II heart failure. J Am Coll Cardiol 2007;49(16):
1696–704.

[119] Masoudi FA, Inzucchi SE, Wang Y, et al. Thiazolidinediones, metformin, and outcomes in older
patients with diabetes and heart failure: an observational study. Circulation 2005;111(5):583–90.

[120] Eurich DT, Majumdar SR, McAlister FA, et al.
Improved clinical outcomes associated with met-
formin in patients with diabetes and heart failure.
Diabetes Care 2005;28(10):2345–51.

[121] Nichols GA, Koro CE, Gullion CM, et al. The incidence of congestive heart failure associated with
antidiabetic therapies. Diabetes Metab Res Rev
2005;21(1):51–7.

[122] Schimmack G, Defronzo RA, Musi N. AMP-acti-
vated protein kinase: role in metabolism and

therapeutic implications. Diabetes Obes Metab 2006;8(6):591–602.

[123] Prepoli MF, Davos C, Francis DP, et al. Exercise training meta-analysis of trials in patients with chronic heart failure (ExTra MATCH). BMJ 2004;328:189–95.

[124] Lavie CJ, Milani RV. Obesity and cardiovascular disease: the Hippocrates paradox. J Am Coll Cardiol 2003;42:677–9.

[125] Lautamaki R, Airaksinin HE, Seppanen M, et al. Rosiglitazone improves myocardial glucose uptake in patients with type 2 diabetes and coronary artery disease: a 16 week randomized, double-blind, placebo-controlled study. Diabetes 2005;54(9): 2787–94.

[126] Sokos GG, Nikolaidis LA, Mankad S, et al. Glucagon-like peptide-1 infusion improves left ventricular ejection fraction and functional status in patients with chronic heart failure. J Card Fail 2006;12(9):694–9.

[127] Thrainsdottir I, Malmberg K, Olsson A, et al. Initial experience with GLP-1 treatment on metabolic control and myocardial function in patients with type 2 diabetes mellitus and heart failure. Diab Vasc Dis Res 2004;1(1):40–3.

[128] Bybee KA, Das S, O'Keefe JH. The rationale and indications for angiotensin receptor blockers in heart failure. Heart Fail Clin 2006;2(1):81–8.

[129] Hodroj W, Legedz L, Foudi N, et al. Increased insulin-stimulated expression of arterial angiotensinogen and angiotensin type 1 receptor in patients with type 2 diabetes mellitus and atheroma. Arterioscler Thromb Vasc Biol 2007; 27(3):525–31.

[130] Katz AM. Heart failure: a hemodynamic disorder complicated by maladaptive proliferative responses. J Cell Mol Med 2003;7(1):1–10.

[131] Sharpe N, Smith H, Murphy J, et al. Early prevention of left ventricular dysfunction after myocardial infarction with angiotensin-converting enzyme inhibition. Lancet 1991;337(8746):872–6.

[132] Moyé LA, Pfeffer MA, Wun CC, et al. Uniformity of captopril benefit in the SAVE study: subgroup analysis. Survival and Ventricular Enlargement Study. Eur Heart J 1994;15(Suppl B):2–8.

[133] Zuanetti G, Latini R, Maggioni AP, et al. Effect of the ACE inhibitor lisinopril on mortality in diabetic patients with acute myocardial infarction: data from the GISSI-3 study. Circulation 1997;96(12): 4239–45.

[134] Gustafsson I, Torp-Pedersen C, Kober L, et al. Effect of the angiotensin-converting enzyme inhibitor trandolapril on diabetic mortality and morbidity in diabetic patients with left ventricular dysfunction after acute myocardial infarction. Trace Study Group. J Am Coll Cardiol 1999;34(1):83–9.

[135] Brenner BM, Cooper ME, de Zeeuw D, et al. RENAAL Study Investigators. Effects of losartan on renal and cardiovascular outcomes in patients with type 2 diabetes and nephropathy. N Engl J Med 2001;345(12):861–9.

[136] Granger CB, McMurray JJ, Yusuf S, et al. CHARM Investigators and Committees. Effects of candesartan in patients with chronic heart failure and reduced left-ventricular systolic function intolerant to angiotensin-converting enzyme inhibitors: the CHARM-Alternative trial. Lancet 2003; 362(9386):772–6.

[137] McMurray JJ, Ostergren J, Swedberg K, et al. CHARM Investigators and Committees. Effects of candesartan in patients with chronic heart failure and reduced left-ventricular systolic function taking angiotensin-converting enzyme inhibitors: the CHARM-Added trial. Lancet 2003;362(9386): 767–71.

[138] Yusuf S, Ostergren JB, Gerstein HC, et al. Candesartan in Heart Failure-Assessment of Reduction in Mortality and Morbidity Program Investigators. Effects of candesartan on the development of a new diagnosis of diabetes mellitus in patients with heart failure. Circulation 2005; 112(1):48–53.

[139] Cohn JN, Tognoni G. Valsartan Heart Failure Trial Investigators. A randomized trial of the angiotensin-receptor blocker valsartan in chronic heart failure. N Engl J Med 2001;345(23):1667–75.

[140] Brown NJ. Aldosterone and end-organ damage. Curr Opin Nephrol Hypertens 2005;14(3):235–41.

[141] Pitt B, Zannad F, Remme WJ, et al. The effect of spironolactone on morbidity and mortality in patients with severe heart failure: Randomized Aldactone Evaluation Study Investigators. N Engl J Med 1999;341(10):709–17.

[142] Pitt B, Remme W, Zannad F, et al. Eplerenone Post-Acute Myocardial Infarction Heart Failure Efficacy and Survival Study Investigators. Eplerenone, a selective aldosterone blocker, in patients with left ventricular dysfunction after myocardial infarction. N Engl J Med 2003;348(14):1309–21.

[143] Juurlink DN, Mamdani MM, Lee DS, et al. Rates of hyperkalemia after publication of the Randomized Aldactone Evaluation Study. N Engl J Med 2004;351(6):543–51.

[144] Large DM, Carr PH, Laing I, et al. Hyperkalaemia in diabetes mellitus: potential hazards of coexisting hyporeninaemic hypoaldosteronism. Postgrad Med J 1984;60(703):370–3.

[145] Haas SJ, Vos T, Gilbert RE, et al. Are beta-blockers as efficacious in patients with diabetes mellitus as in patients without diabetes mellitus who have chronic heart failure? A meta-analysis of large-scale clinical trials. Am Heart J 2003;146(5): 848–53.

[146] Bakris GL, Fonseca V, Katholi RE, et al. GEMINI Investigators. Metabolic effects of carvedilol vs metoprolol in patients with type 2 diabetes mellitus and hypertension: a randomized controlled trial. JAMA 2004;292(18):2227–36.

ELSEVIER
SAUNDERS

Cardiol Clin 25 (2007) 539–551

CARDIOLOGY
CLINICS

Pharmacologic Therapy for Acute Heart Failure

W. H. Wilson Tang, MD, FACC, FAHA

Cleveland Clinic, Cleveland, OH, USA

Existing therapies for acute heart failure syndrome (AHFS) have three main therapeutic goals: (1) to relieve congestion, (2) to reduce abnormal loading conditions, and (3) to improve myocardial contractility and relaxation. This article reviews the evolution of pharmacologic therapy in treating AHFS, with special emphasis on knowledge gained from results of recent clinical trials (Table 1), as well as a discussion on the limitations of current therapies.

Diuretic therapy—targeting congestion

The most significant advancement in our understanding of treatment patterns and clinical outcomes in the contemporary management of AHFS stems from insight gained from the Acute Decompensated Heart Failure National Registry (ADHERE) [1]. This large nationwide survey of AHFS admissions highlights several contemporary management strategies for AHFS. For example, diuretic therapy remains the mainstay of pharmacologic therapy in congestive states of AHFS, with over 85% of admitted patients receiving diuretic therapy as their primary therapeutic intervention. In the majority of patients, loop diuretics are the only intravenous intervention during admission.

The goal of diuretic therapy is to remove excess volume accumulated in the setting of heart failure, usually resulting from a combination of neurohormonal overactivation, excess sodium intake from dietary noncompliance, drug noncompliance, and changes in underlying medical conditions (eg, arrhythmia, renal insufficiency, myocardial ischemia). The biggest challenge in the use of diuretic therapy has been accurately defining and assessing

the appropriate "targets" of therapy. Most clinicians use a combination of clinical and self-reported signs and symptoms to gauge the appropriate discharge timing, and diuretic therapy can often achieve success in relieving congestive symptoms in the majority of admitted patients.

Currently, there is no general agreement regarding guidance from biomarkers or other noninvasive physiologic measures that can provide a reliable objective assessment of intravascular volume status. Although promising and commonly used as a surrogate for disease severity in heart failure, plasma levels of B-type natriuretic peptide (BNP) may not be as reliable in the assessment of volume status in AHFS because changes in levels may not accurately reflect changes in hemodynamics [2] or blood volume [3]. Nevertheless, preliminary data suggest that a BNP-guided strategy may provide some benefit when compared with lack of BNP guidance [4,5], at least in the acute setting, and confirmatory trials are currently ongoing.

Loop diuretics

Loop diuretic therapy (furosemide, torsemide, bumetanide) is perhaps one of the most commonly prescribed yet least researched pharmacotherapies for AHFS. These drugs inhibit the reabsorption of sodium and chloride in the ascending limb of the loop of Henle by blocking the $Na^+/K^+/2Cl^-$ transporter, thereby removing salt with accompanying water. It is customary to consider the overall equivalence in efficacy between different loop diuretic drugs in their intravenous forms, even though their bioavailabilities and their protein-binding affinities may differ in their respective oral formulations [6].

Dosing is usually empirical, in part, due to the approval and broad adoption of diuretic therapy before the era of evidence-based medicine and randomized clinical trials. Most dosing strategies use an initial intravenous bolus administration,

Dr. Tang is a consultant for NovaCardiac Inc., Astellas Pharma Inc., and Biosite Inc., and has received research grant from Abbott Diagnostics Inc.

E-mail address: tangw@ccf.org

Table 1
Contemporary multicenter randomized controlled trials for vasoactive drugs in patients with acute heart failure syndrome

Drug	Trial	Sample size	Primary endpoint	Results
Diuretics/aquaretics				
Tolvaptan	EVEREST [19,20]	4133	All-cause mortality and cardiovascular death or hospitalization	No effect on long-term mortality or heart failure hospitalizations but improved signs/symptoms (day 7)
Vasodilators				
Nesiritide	VMAC [33]	489	Change in PCWP and dyspnea at 3 h	Significant improvement in both endpoints, no improvement in renal function, hospitalization, or death
Ularitide	SIRIUS-2 [40]	221	Hemodynamic changes	Dose-dependent improvement in hemodynamic parameters, without higher adverse clinical events
Tezosentan	RITZ-1 [44]	666	Dyspnea at 24 h	Worsening renal function with tezosentan
	RITZ-2 [43]	285	Hemodynamic changes	Significant improvement in hemodynamics
	VERITAS [45]	1435	Dyspnea at 24 h, and death/worsening heart failure at 7 d	Significant improvement in hemodynamics, but terminated early due to futility
Inotropic drugs				
Milrinone	OPTIME-CHF [54]	949	Days hospitalized for cardiovascular cause at 60 d	No difference in events, but higher risk of hypotension and atrial arrhythmia for milrinone group
Levosimendan	LIDO [56]	203	Hemodynamic changes	Improved 180-d mortality
	REVIVE-1 [59]	100	Clinical outcomes	Improved adverse outcomes at 24 h and 5 d
	REVIVE-2 [60]	600	Composite clinical presentation	Improved composite clinical endpoint Neutral effects on 90-d mortality despite reduced BNP
	SURVIVE [61]	1327	180-d survival	No differences in 180-d mortality despite reduced BNP versus dobutamine

Abbreviations: BNP, B-type natriuretic peptide; d, day; h, hour; PCWP, pulmonary capillary wedge pressures.

although continuous loop diuretic infusions have been explored in several small and uncontrolled studies [7,8] as well as a recent Cochrane database review [9]. These data provide some reassurance that steady infusion of loop diuretics may provide effective diuresis beyond what can be achieved by bolus loop diuretics and with lower risks of side effects including ototoxicity and azotemia. As outlined in the latest Heart Failure Society of America (HFSA) guidelines, adverse effects of intravenous loop diuretics such as renal dysfunction, electrolyte abnormalities, and symptomatic

hypotension should be carefully monitored [10]. It is also clear that these adverse effects are dose and route dependent [11] and may be related to an excessively rapid reduction in intravascular volume; however, the exact underlying mechanisms are likely complex. Sometimes loop diuretics can be combined with thiazides or other diuretic drugs to augment their diuretic and natriuretic effects in severe volume overload or refractory congestion, although at a higher risk of adverse effects [12].

Two of the three most important prognostic determinants for in-hospital mortality for AHFS include measures of renal function [13]. There is an increasing recognition that intravenous loop diuretics are notorious in creating overzealous diuresis and natriuresis within a short duration of drug action, leading to intravascular volume depletion and subsequent azotemia, hypotension, and renal insufficiency. Several studies have suggested that up to one third of patients admitted for AHFS may experience worsening renal function (defined as absolute increase in serum creatinine ≥ 0.3–0.5 mg/dL [14]) as well as electrolyte imbalances. There is also reason to believe that, in some situations, overzealous loop diuretic therapy may lead to salt and volume depletion and diminished natriuresis, allowing the potential benefits of concomitant hypertonic saline for more effective diuresis [15].

Vasopressin receptor antagonists

Arginine vasopressin has long been recognized as an up-regulated neurohormonal system regulating water and salt balance. With the primary goal being to remove water rather than salt, non-peptide antagonists targeting vasopressin receptors have been explored as "aquaretic" agents blocking the effects of vasopressin at the V_2 receptors in the collecting duct of the kidney. Tolvaptan has been the most widely studied agent, and both tolvaptan and lixivaptan have demonstrated a dose-dependent aquaretic effect accompanying weight loss without renal compromise [16,17]. Nevertheless, the clinical benefits of these "vaptan" drugs have yet to be realized. For example, long-term tolvaptan use was not related to any reversal in cardiac remodeling, an important surrogate for improved outcomes in heart failure [18]. Furthermore, despite a slight short-term improvement in symptomatic relief, the recent pivotal Efficacy of Vasopressin Antagonism in Heart Failure Outcome Study with Tolvaptan (EVEREST) trial did not show any significant long-term mortality benefit with oral tolvaptan over standard diuretic therapy when given during admission (Fig. 1) [19,20]. Hence, finding a cost-effective superior drug to complement or substitute loop diuretics remains exceedingly challenging.

Vasodilator therapy—targeting abnormal loading

Another interesting observation from ADHERE was the overall hemodynamic profile of patients presenting with AHFS [21]. Although few patients underwent cardiac catheterization to fully appreciate their underlying cardiac physiology, it

was observed that over 90% of patients had relatively preserved blood pressure (ie, systolic blood pressure >90 mm Hg). In fact, what is more surprising was that over half of the admissions documented a systolic blood pressure greater than 140 mm Hg. These findings confirm that AHFS is a problem of vascular insufficiency (with associated abnormal relaxation) rather than primarily an incremental impairment of myocardial contractility. With the availability of vasodilator drugs in clinical development, there has been a recent resurgence of interest in the appropriate use of vasodilator therapy in AHFS.

Nitroprusside and nitroglycerin

Sodium nitroprusside and nitroglycerin have been used in less than 5% of all patients presenting with AHFS in ADHERE [21]. Both drugs are vasodilators that exert their actions via conversion to nitric oxide, although nitroglycerin is primarily a venodilator whereas sodium nitroprusside is considered to have arterial vasodilatory effects. These therapies may also have differential effects on different vascular beds, although much of this data has been historical and derived from small mechanistic studies without long-term outcomes. Sodium nitroprusside and nitroglycerin are still supported in the latest guidelines despite a paucity of contemporary clinical evidence [10,22].

Sodium nitroprusside has highly favorable hemodynamic effects in patients with refractory heart failure [23,24], especially in terms of its ability to augment the cardiac index and lower peripheral vascular resistance [25] as well as improve left atrial and left ventricular function [26]. Nevertheless, a large randomized trial conducted in 812 patients with post-infarction left ventricular failure observed no significant differences in short- or long-term mortality and instead found concerns of increased risk when used within the first 9 hours of infarction [27]. Case reports of thiocyanate toxicity and the need for close hemodynamic monitoring have also hampered enthusiasm for its use.

In a head-to-head comparison, patients treated with high-dose nitroglycerin plus low-dose furosemide had lower rates of death, mechanical ventilation, and myocardial infarction when compared with patients treated with low-dose nitroglycerin plus high-dose furosemide [28]. Despite a perceived lower risk profile for toxicity and its ability to lower intracardiac filling pressures [25], intravenous

542 TANG

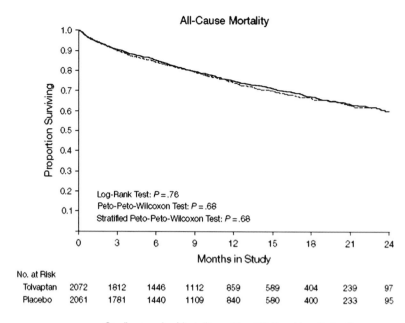

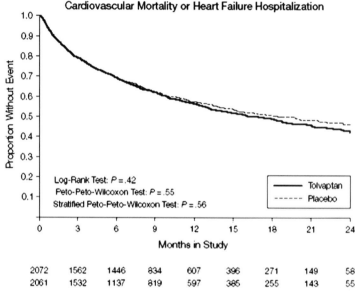

Fig. 1. Kaplan-Meier survival curve for tolvaptan in AHFS. (*From* Konstam MA, Gheorghiade M, Burnett JC Jr, et al. Effects of oral tolvaptan in patients hospitalized for worsening heart failure: the EVEREST Outcome Trial. JAMA 2007;297(12):1323; with permission.)

nitroglycerin has limitations including the development of tolerance with continuous use [29].

Natriuretic peptides

Natriuretic peptides have emerged as potentially useful therapeutic agents in the treatment of patients with AHFS. Three compounds that are analogues of different types of natriuretic peptides have been developed and used in different countries. Nesiritide is the intravenous form of the recombinant human BNP approved in the United States, which has been observed to provide a dose-dependent reduction in intracardiac pressures and improvement in heart failure symptoms [30]. Despite being classified as a natriuretic peptide, nesiritide has not been associated with significant diuresis in mechanistic studies [31] and has primarily been considered a vasodilator that can improve hemodynamics [32]. Nesiritide was compared with intravenous nitroglycerin in the Vasodilation in the Management of Acute Congestive Heart Failure (VMAC) trial, which randomized 489 AHFS patients to either treatment strategy in comparison with placebo for 24 hours. The mean change in pulmonary capillary wedge pressure (PCWP) at 3 hours was −5.8 mm Hg for nesiritide, −3.8 mm Hg for nitroglycerin, and −2 mm Hg in placebo ($P < .03$). This improvement corresponded to improved patients' self-perception of dyspnea at 3 hours (but not to dyspnea scores) [33]. In the VMAC trial, there were no significant differences in 6-month mortality rates between the nesiritide group and the nitroglycerin group (25% versus 21%). Interestingly, in the subgroup of patients who did not undergo catheterization (n = 243), nesiritide had no significant effect on dyspnea when compared with placebo but significantly improved dyspnea when compared with nitroglycerin at 24 hours.

This relatively small but significant difference in hemodynamic profile has led to much debate regarding the potential advantage of nesiritide over nitroglycerin to justify its relatively high cost. Further scrutiny using meta-analysis techniques has added concern regarding its long-term safety profile. In a review of a series of publications and study results, nesiritide significantly increased the risk of worsening renal function (defined as an increase in serum creatinine > 0.5 mg/dL) when compared with a control (relative risk, 1.52 for non-inotropic control [$P = .003$] versus 1.54 for any control [$P = .001$]) [34]; however, subsequent prospective studies have not yet replicated this risk [35,36]. Furthermore, a pooled analysis of three randomized controlled trials revealed a trend toward a higher 30-day mortality rate in the nesiritide group when compared with the non-inotrope control group (35 [7.2%] of 485 versus 15 [4.0%] of 377 patients; risk ratio, 1.74 [$P = .059$]) [37]. Both the original studies and the meta-analyses had limitations in addressing long-term risks versus benefits and did not account for the heterogeneity of the patient population as well as concurrent and subsequent interventions. Nevertheless, when analyzed with longer-term follow-up, a 180-day mortality risk associated with nesiritide was not apparent (Fig. 2) [38].

Although a controversial debate followed the publication of these meta-analyses, enthusiasm over the use of nesiritide is diminishing [39], and its use will be dependent on the ongoing 7000-patient ASCEND-HF (Acute Study of Clinical Effectiveness of Nesiritide in Decompensated Heart Failure) outcomes trial to re-establish its role in AHFS therapy.

Carperitide (recombinant atrial natriuretic peptide) has been approved in Japan, but its clinical development has been discontinued in the United States. In contrast, ularitide has been evaluated in a phase II study (SIRIUS-II, or Safety and Efficacy of an Intravenous Placebo-Controlled Randomized Infusion of Ularitide), in which a dose-dependent improvement in hemodynamics was observed with ularitide [40]. This effect was accompanied by no significant difference in renal function or adverse event rates between treatment and control groups. Ularitide is currently undergoing clinical development in Europe (phase III studies).

Other vasodilators

Following the success of targeting neurohormonal up-regulation as a therapeutic strategy in chronic heart failure, several neurohormonal systems demonstrating vasoconstrictive properties have been identified as potential therapeutic targets for AHFS. Intravenous angiotensin-converting enzymes have not been evaluated after potential detrimental consequences were associated with the early use of enalaprilat in the post-infarction setting [41]. Endothelin is another vasoconstrictor system that is operative in the setting of heart failure and pulmonary hypertension. In AHFS, the intravenous endothelin receptor antagonist tezosentan has been found to relieve signs and symptoms and improve hemodynamics and outcomes in small mechanistic studies [42–44]; however, the large pivotal study, VERITAS (Value of Endothelin Receptor Inhibition with Tezosentan in Acute heart failure Study) [45], was terminated in late 2005 due to futility despite producing the expected hemodynamic responses. This finding highlights the challenge of appropriate patient selection for vasodilator therapy in AHFS, and the difficulty of balancing the benefits of afterload reduction with the risks of overzealous vasodilation. Intravenous hydralazine has been used in AHFS as a vasodilator drug. In patients with refractory heart failure requiring inotropic therapy, the addition of hydralazine has

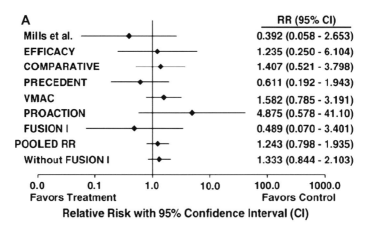

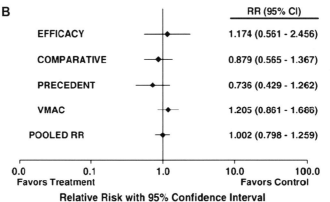

Fig. 2. Pooled analysis of 30-day (*A*) and 180-day (*B*) relative risk for mortality for nesiritide versus control. (*From* Arora RR, Venkatesh PK, Molnar J. Short and long-term mortality with nesiritide. Am Heart J 2006;152(6): 1086–7; with permission).

been found to be effective in facilitating withdrawal of dobutamine therapy [46].

Inotropic therapy—targeting impaired myocardial contractility or relaxation

Inotropic therapy has the benefit of rapidly improving adverse hemodynamic profiles, particularly in the setting of low cardiac output; however, no inotropic therapy (or inodilator) to date can avoid the increase in oxygen demand as well as the promotion of intracellular calcium accumulation leading to potential arrhythmic complications. In the ADHERE database, approximately 14% of patients were treated with inotropic agents (more accurately described as "inodilators"), and approximately 2% were discharged on chronic infusion therapy with either dobutamine or milrinone [21]. Similar usage rates were found in OPTIMIZE-HF (Organized Program to Initiate Life-saving

Treatment in Hospitalized Patients with Heart Failure) enrollees with systolic blood pressure less than 120 mm Hg [47]. Patients who received inotropic agents during their admission had unadjusted in-hospital mortality rates as high as 14% [48].

There have also been indicators that the use of inotropic therapy may reflect either a bias in patients who presented with more advanced heart failure or even a predilection of use based on the individual physician's discretion. In a recently published sub-analysis of the ESCAPE (Evaluation Study of Congestive Heart Failure and Pulmonary Artery Catheterization Effectiveness) trial, propensity-score adjusted multivariable risk factor models for mortality were not statistically significant for vasodilators (n = 75, hazard ratio [HR] =1.39, P = .403) but were significant for inotropic drugs (n = 133, HR = 2.14, P = .024) and the need for both drugs (n = 47, HR = 4.81, P < .001) [49]. Similar results were found for risk-adjusted

6-month mortality and re-hospitalization models (Fig. 3). Although hemodynamic and renal parameters are important predictors of vasoactive drug use, individual sites have a large influence on the decision to use vasodilators or inotropic drugs, reflecting subjective biases and practice variations present in the clinical setting [49].

Catecholamines

Continuous infusions of dobutamine and dopamine aim to augment myocardial contractility via direct stimulation of β_1-adrenergic receptors. Interestingly, short-term infusion of catecholamines (dobutamine or dopamine) has not been thoroughly examined in randomized clinical trials, although small series have demonstrated improvements in heart failure symptoms and cardiac contractility with dobutamine infusions [50]. Studies have indirectly shown that dobutamine infusion is associated with significantly increased rates of arrhythmic events when compared with nesiritide [51] and may be associated with increased long-term mortality risk [52]. Dobutamine and dopamine are currently used in patients with advanced refractory heart failure to relieve symptoms and to improve end-organ function in low-output states in the urgent setting, although their long-term safety profile remains somewhat unresolved. In patients receiving intermediate- to long-term infusion while awaiting cardiac transplantation, clinical event rates were comparable between dobutamine and milrinone [53].

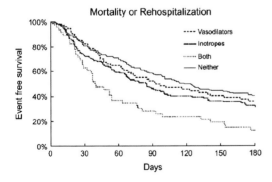

Fig. 3. Kaplan-Meier survival curve for freedom from death or re-hospitalization by intravenous vasoactive medication use. (*From* Elkayam U, Tasissa G, Binanay C, et al. Use and impact of inotropes and vasodilator therapy in hospitalized patients with severe heart failure. Am Heart J 2007;153(1):102; with permission).

Phosphodiesterase inhibitors

Milrinone and amrinone are the two drugs that have been approved for AHFS, but the latter is seldom used due to risks of bone marrow suppression. Short-term use of intravenous milrinone has been evaluated in the Outcomes of Prospective Trial of Intravenous Milrinone for Exacerbations of Chronic Heart Failure (OPTIME-CHF) [54]. In that study, routine use of intravenous milrinone compared with placebo as an adjunct to standard therapy in patients with AHFS resulted in no statistically significant differences in the number of days hospitalized for cardiovascular causes [54]; however, more patients in the milrinone group had sustained hypotension and arrhythmia, and milrinone may even be deleterious in patients with ischemic cardiomyopathy [55]. Patients enrolled in OPTIME-CHF did not necessarily require inotropic support.

Levosimendan

Levosimendan has a unique dual mechanism of action. First, the ability of levosimendan to increase inotropy via increasing the sensitivity of cardiac troponin C to intracellular ionized calcium without increasing myocardial oxygen consumption has earned its classification as a "calcium sensitizer." In addition, the ability to facilitate potassium-ATP channel opening may provide additional beneficial vasodilatory effects. Nevertheless, there is ongoing debate regarding whether levosimendan is a unique agent or whether it is still simply another phosphodiesterase inhibitor. Early studies using levosimendan have provided support in treating decompensated patients in the AHFS (when compared with dobutamine) [56] and in post-infarction settings (when compared with placebo) [57]. There are also preliminary reports in an open-label trial that suggest using levosimendan may provide mortality and symptomatic benefits over placebo and dobutamine [58,59], leading to its approval in some countries outside the United States.

Recently, two large, double-blind, prospective, randomized control trials that evaluated the efficacy of levosimendan in AHFS patients have provided further support for additional benefits of levosimendan over standard therapy, although the significance of these results is under intense debate. The second Randomized Multicenter Evaluation of Intravenous Levosimendan Efficacy (REVIVE-2) demonstrated that intravenous levosimendan was more likely to be associated with clinical improvement using a composite scale when used in addition to standard therapy [60].

The addition of levosimendan to standard therapy resulted in lower plasma BNP values, a shorter duration of admission, and better relief of symptoms when compared with standard therapy alone; however, the number of deaths was greater in the levosimendan arm (35 versus 45 deaths at 90 days), albeit, not statistically significant. In contrast, in the Survival Of Patients With Acute Heart Failure In Need Of Intravenous Inotropic Support (SURVIVE) study, a head-to-head comparison between levosimendan and dobutamine found no significant differences in 180-day mortality between the two treatment arms (26% versus 28%, respectively, $P = .401$) [61]. After 5 days of treatment, BNP decreased by 46% in those who received levosimendan compared with only 13% in the dobutamine group [61]; however, the use of levosimendan failed to meet its primary goal of reducing mortality by 25% at 6 months (Fig. 4). Based on these two contemporary studies involving up to 2000 AHFS subjects, levosimendan administration can provide short-term relief of symptoms and an improved clinical course when compared with placebo or to dobutamine. All-cause mortality was not statistically significant between the groups, although it was numerically greater when compared with that for the placebo group and lower when compared with that for the dobutamine group. During the 3- to 6-month follow-up period, levosimendan was associated with an increased incidence of atrial fibrillation and ventricular tachycardia (the latter only when compared with placebo and not with

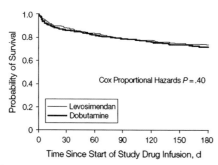

No. at Risk

Levosimendan	664	608	586		525		462
Dobutamine	663	596	568		519		454

Fig. 4. Kaplan-Meier survival curve for levosimendan versus dobutamine in AHFS. (*From* Mebazaa A, Nieminen MS, Packer M, et al. Levosimendan versus dobutamine for patients with acute decompensated heart failure: the SURVIVE Randomized Trial. JAMA 2007;297(17):1885; with permission. Copyright © 2007, American Medical Association. All rights reserved.)

dobutamine). Currently, levosimendan is approved in Europe but not in the United States.

Current challenges in clinical development of pharmacologic therapy for acute heart failure syndrome

Appropriate trial designs

There are major challenges in current pharmacologic approaches to AHFS, in part, due to the lack of reliable and acceptable trial designs that can definitively identify effective therapies, as well as confounding factors beyond direct drug effects (eg, concomitant therapies, lack of effective blinding, and adverse effects due to a lack of reliable therapeutic targets). Large-scale randomized trials are few and challenging, and many reported trials (particularly ones that demonstrate effectiveness of a therapy) are unblinded.

Appropriate therapeutic targets

The fundamental challenge of AHFS drug development is the lack of understanding of appropriate therapeutic targets. Although great strides have been made in understanding the pathophysiology of chronic stable heart failure, one of the biggest challenges in understanding the role of pharmacologic therapy in AHFS is the inability to distinguish different biologic processes that are being affected. Instead of defining an abnormal physiology, most definitions of AHFS describe the need for a change in location of care (hospital, emergency department, urgent clinic visits) in response to a rapid change in the constellation of signs and symptoms secondary to an abnormal cardiac function (eg, worsening dyspnea, edema, orthopnea).

Appropriate study population

Defining the appropriate study population has been the single most important challenge in AHFS trials. AHFS does not yet have a universally accepted definition, in part, because limited clinical measurements can clearly define the disease process. Relying on signs and symptoms of clinical presentation can be analogous to using chest pain for inclusion criteria for antithrombotic drug trials in acute coronary syndromes. Furthermore, the large majority of AHFS trials continue to focus on impaired left ventricular systolic function (systolic heart failure) as part of inclusion criteria, ignoring the fact that at least half of all AHFS patients may present with a preserved left ventricular ejection fraction. Even the ongoing clinical trials may lack a consistent characterization of AHFS using biomarkers such as natriuretic peptide testing or through hemodynamic assessment due to logistic constraints. It is likely that, in the future, biomarkers will have an important role in patient selection for AHFS therapies. Biomarkers may even guide cardiologists in distinguishing patients who may or may not be appropriate for a specific intervention. For example, providing a cut-off value for plasma BNP levels may allow effective exclusion of subjects below that cut-off, whereas higher BNP levels may be able to identify patients with a higher risk for adverse clinical events, thereby reducing the sample size of the trial.

Appropriate drug comparator

The appropriate drug comparator is always a debate. Due to the lack of evidence-based guidelines and consensus, treatment for AHFS may vary considerably. For drugs that relieve congestion, adequate dosing or confounding due to the standard of care (intravenous loop diuretics) may influence the true effects of the study drug when congestive signs and symptoms are the endpoints. The same is true for vasodilator therapies, in which overzealous or prolonged diuretic therapy before or during the study period may lead to a greater propensity for developing adverse events such as azotemia or hypotension. In inodilator therapy, the potential benefit of a study drug may be magnified by the perceived risk of dobutamine therapy as a comparator.

Appropriate timing and dosing of intervention

The timing and dosing of the intervention can also have an impact on the outcomes studied. In EVEREST, the lack of significant effects with oral tolvaptan has been attributed, in part, to the potential delayed administration of the study drug; powerful diuretic effects of intravenous loop diuretics may have already ameliorated congestive symptoms. Hence, the protective effects a drug may add to current pharmacologic strategies must take into account the way AHFS is currently treated. The decision to use a drug in a fixed-dose versus titrating-dose manner is dependent on the perceived drug effects and the potential adverse effects of the intervention. As an example, the large variability of responses to vasodilatory therapy provides challenges to standardizing a treatment regimen in study design.

Appropriate endpoints

Identifying an appropriate and acceptable endpoint can also be a challenge. Most early clinical studies are unblinded, mainly because they are based on achieving and maintaining hemodynamic targets as a reliable surrogate outcome for AHFS. The VMAC study is a good example [33] in which a statistically significant improvement in the primary endpoint (change in PCWP or dyspnea in 3 hours) can be challenged by concerns of long-term benefits and resistance to broad adoption due to high expenses. Similarly, a statistically significant drop in BNP shortly after admission did not translate into better long-term outcomes in SURVIVE for levosimendan over dobutamine [61]. There is an increasing demand to demonstrate a reduction in re-hospitalizations and long-term morbidity and mortality for a new drug intervention to be acceptable. Based on results from clinical trials for vasopressin receptor antagonists and ultrafiltration strategies, the ability of a drug to reduce body weight in the setting of volume overload may be an attractive surrogate for improving long-term clinical outcomes. In contrast, although logical by deduction, the ability of an intervention to preserve renal function has yet to directly translate into improvement of long-term outcomes in the setting of AHFS.

Future perspectives

Several promising drugs are currently undergoing clinical development for the treatment of AHFS. These studies have all adopted the large-scale, multicenter clinical trial approach, although many of the aforementioned challenges are still unresolved as reflected by the vast array of selection criteria as well as primary and secondary endpoints.

Following the relatively neutral results on long-term outcomes for tolvaptan, many V_2-specific (eg, lixivaptan) as well as dual V_{1a}/V_2 vasopressin receptor antagonists (eg, conivaptan) have been reassessed in regard to their potential for incremental benefits in the treatment of AHFS. Nevertheless, a Phase III study on lixivaptan is commencing (BALANCE). However, renal preservation remains an important and likely viable therapeutic target; a novel class of drugs can improve the renal blood flow and augment sodium excretion via the blockade of adenosine A_1 receptors. A large prospective trial program is currently ongoing to evaluate the role of KW-3902 in the preservation of renal function as well as reducing adverse clinical events in de novo admissions of AHFS patients (PROTECT-1 and PROTECT-2) as well as those developing worsening renal insufficiency (REACH-UP). Other adenosine A_1 receptor antagonists, such as SLV320 or BG-9928 (Biogen Idec), are also undergoing early phase development.

Several clinical trials are also ongoing to explore and define the role of vasoactive therapies in patients with AHFS. To refine understanding of the safety and efficacy of nesiritide, a large, worldwide, multicenter, randomized controlled trial has been initiated (ASCEND-HF). This study is one of the largest AHFS trials conducted to date and will explore both short-term and long-term effects of intravenous nesiritide in the setting of AHFS. Other vasodilators, including ularitide, will also be tested in a similar manner, and alternative routes of delivery will be explored (eg, subcutaneous infusion or targeted renal therapy by direct catheter-based delivery to the renal arteries).

Although inodilators have fallen out of favor as the primary strategy for AHFS, they still provide temporary (or even permanent) support for selected patients with advanced heart failure when therapeutic options are limited. Novel compounds continue to emerge, such as istaroxime (an inhibitor of Na^+/K^+-ATPase that increases SERCA2a activity) and specific cardiac myosin activators (eg, CK-1827452). Many of these novel inotropic drugs will likely be used as chronic therapy rather than in an acute "salvage" approach as seen in some AHFS patients.

Summary

Over the past decades, many heroic attempts have been made to address the challenges facing the care of patients with AHFS. The central objective in treating AHFS is largely based on reducing the congestive state. The underlying reasons leading to congestion may not be obvious, and the optimal balance of cardiac, vascular, and renal alterations necessary to maintain minimal symptoms and maximal survival has yet to be established. This failure can be explained by the ongoing lack of "positive" clinical trials in AHFS that can unequivocally demonstrate the ability of a pharmacologic agent to achieve a universally acceptable outcome.

As more extant and novel pharmacologic strategies advance into clinical development, equally important are the parallel efforts to identify the best ways to use existing drugs and devices to prevent the progression to AHFS or to guide therapy following the identification of AHFS.

References

[1] Fonarow GC. The Acute Decompensated Heart Failure National Registry (ADHERE): opportunities to improve care of patients hospitalized with acute decompensated heart failure. Rev Cardiovasc Med 2003;4(Suppl 7):S21–30.

[2] O'Neill JO, Bott-Silverman CE, McRae AT 3rd, et al. B-type natriuretic peptide levels are not a surrogate marker for invasive hemodynamics during management of patients with severe heart failure. Am Heart J 2005;149(2):363–9.

[3] James KB, Troughton RW, Feldschuh J, et al. Blood volume and brain natriuretic peptide in congestive heart failure: a pilot study. Am Heart J 2005;150: 984.e1–984.e6.

[4] Jourdain P, Jondeau G, Funck F, et al. Plasma brain natriuretic peptide-guided therapy to improve outcome in heart failure: the STARS-BNP Multicenter Study. J Am Coll Cardiol 2007;49(16): 1733–9.

[5] Moe GW, Howlett J, Januzzi JL, et al. N-terminal pro-B-type natriuretic peptide testing improves the management of patients with suspected acute heart failure: primary results of the Canadian prospective randomized multicenter IMPROVE-CHF study. Circulation 2007;115(24):3103–10.

[6] Vargo DL, Kramer WG, Black PK, et al. Bioavailability, pharmacokinetics, and pharmacodynamics of torsemide and furosemide in patients with congestive heart failure. Clin Pharmacol Ther 1995;57(6): 601–9.

[7] van Meyel JJ, Smits P, Dormans T, et al. Continuous infusion of furosemide in the treatment of patients with congestive heart failure and diuretic resistance. J Intern Med 1994;235(4):329–34.

[8] Dormans TP, van Meyel JJ, Gerlag PG, et al. Diuretic efficacy of high dose furosemide in severe heart failure: bolus injection versus continuous infusion. J Am Coll Cardiol 1996;28(2):376–82.

[9] Salvador DR, Rey NR, Ramos GC, et al. Continuous infusion versus bolus injection of loop diuretics in congestive heart failure. Cochrane Database Syst Rev 2005;(3):CD003178.

[10] Heart Failure Society of America. Evaluation and management of patients with acute decompensated heart failure. J Card Fail 2006;12(1):e86–103.

[11] Cotter G, Weissgarten J, Metzkor E, et al. Increased toxicity of high-dose furosemide versus low-dose dopamine in the treatment of refractory congestive heart failure. Clin Pharmacol Ther 1997;62(2): 187–93.

[12] Dormans TP, Gerlag PG, Russel FG, et al. Combination diuretic therapy in severe congestive heart failure. Drugs 1998;55(2):165–72.

[13] Fonarow GC, Adams KF Jr, Abraham WT, et al. Risk stratification for in-hospital mortality in acutely decompensated heart failure: classification and regression tree analysis. JAMA 2005;293(5): 572–80.

[14] Gottlieb SS, Abraham W, Butler J, et al. The prognostic importance of different definitions of worsening renal function in congestive heart failure. J Card Fail 2002;8(3):136–41.

[15] Paterna S, Di Pasquale P, Parrinello G, et al. Changes in brain natriuretic peptide levels and bioelectrical impedance measurements after treatment with high-dose furosemide and hypertonic saline solution versus high-dose furosemide alone in refractory congestive heart failure: a double-blind study. J Am Coll Cardiol 2005;45(12):1997–2003.

[16] Gheorghiade M, Gattis WA, O'Connor CM, et al. Effects of tolvaptan, a vasopressin antagonist, in patients hospitalized with worsening heart failure: a randomized controlled trial. JAMA 2004;291(16): 1963–71.

[17] Abraham WT, Shamshirsaz AA, McFann K, et al. Aquaretic effect of lixivaptan, an oral, non-peptide, selective V2 receptor vasopressin antagonist, in New York Heart Association functional class II and III chronic heart failure patients. J Am Coll Cardiol 2006;47(8):1615–21.

[18] Udelson JE, McGrew FA, Flores E, et al. Multicenter, randomized, double-blind, placebo-controlled study on the effect of oral tolvaptan on left ventricular dilation and function in patients with heart failure and systolic dysfunction. J Am Coll Cardiol 2007;49(22):2151–9.

[19] Gheorghiade M, Konstam MA, Burnett JC Jr, et al. Short-term clinical effects of tolvaptan, an oral vasopressin antagonist, in patients hospitalized for heart failure: the EVEREST clinical status trials. JAMA 2007;297(12):1332–43.

[20] Konstam MA, Gheorghiade M, Burnett JC Jr, et al. Effects of oral tolvaptan in patients hospitalized for worsening heart failure: the EVEREST outcome trial. JAMA 2007;297(12):1319–31.

[21] Adams KF Jr, Fonarow GC, Emerman CL, et al. Characteristics and outcomes of patients hospitalized for heart failure in the United States: rationale, design, and preliminary observations from the first 100,000 cases in the Acute Decompensated Heart Failure National Registry (ADHERE). Am Heart J 2005;149(2):209–16.

[22] Nieminen MS, Bohm M, Cowie MR, et al. Executive summary of the guidelines on the diagnosis and treatment of acute heart failure: the Task Force on Acute Heart Failure of the European Society of Cardiology. Eur Heart J 2005;26(4):384–416.

[23] Guiha NH, Cohn JN, Mikulic E, et al. Treatment of refractory heart failure with infusion of nitroprusside. N Engl J Med 1974;291(12):587–92.

[24] Johnson W, Omland T, Hall C, et al. Neurohormonal activation rapidly decreases after intravenous therapy with diuretics and vasodilators for class IV heart failure. J Am Coll Cardiol 2002; 39(10):1623–9.

[25] Miller RR, Vismara LA, Williams DO, et al. Pharmacological mechanisms for left ventricular unloading in clinical congestive heart failure: differential effects of nitroprusside, phentolamine, and nitroglycerin on cardiac function and peripheral circulation. Circ Res 1976;39(1):127–33.

[26] Capomolla S, Pozzoli M, Opasich C, et al. Dobutamine and nitroprusside infusion in patients with severe congestive heart failure: hemodynamic improvement by discordant effects on mitral regurgitation, left atrial function, and ventricular function. Am Heart J 1997;134(6):1089–98.

[27] Cohn JN, Franciosa JA, Francis GS, et al. Effect of short-term infusion of sodium nitroprusside on mortality rate in acute myocardial infarction complicated by left ventricular failure: results of a Veterans Administration cooperative study. N Engl J Med 1982;306(19):1129–35.

[28] Cotter G, Metzkor E, Kaluski E, et al. Randomised trial of high-dose isosorbide dinitrate plus low-dose furosemide versus high-dose furosemide plus low-dose isosorbide dinitrate in severe pulmonary oedema. Lancet 1998;351(9100):389–93.

[29] Elkayam U, Bitar F, Akhter MW, et al. Intravenous nitroglycerin in the treatment of decompensated heart failure: potential benefits and limitations. J Cardiovasc Pharmacol Ther 2004; 9(4):227–41.

[30] Colucci WS, Elkayam U, Horton DP, et al. Intravenous nesiritide, a natriuretic peptide, in the treatment of decompensated congestive heart failure. Nesiritide Study Group. N Engl J Med 2000;343(4): 246–53.

[31] Wang DJ, Dowling TC, Meadows D, et al. Nesiritide does not improve renal function in patients with chronic heart failure and worsening serum creatinine. Circulation 2004;110(12):1620–5.

[32] Mills RM, LeJemtel TH, Horton DP, et al. Sustained hemodynamic effects of an infusion of nesiritide (human B-type natriuretic peptide) in heart failure: a randomized, double-blind, placebo-controlled clinical trial. Natrecor Study Group. J Am Coll Cardiol 1999;34(1):155–62.

[33] Publication Committee for the VMAC (Vasodilation in the Management of Acute CHF). Intravenous nesiritide vs nitroglycerin for treatment of decompensated congestive heart failure: a randomized controlled trial. JAMA 2002;287:1531–40.

[34] Sackner-Bernstein JD, Skopicki HA, Aaronson KD. Risk of worsening renal function with nesiritide in patients with acutely decompensated heart failure. Circulation 2005;111(12):1487–91.

[35] Yancy CW, Krum H, Massie BM, et al. The Second Follow-up Serial Infusions of Nesiritide (FUSION II) trial for advanced heart failure: study rationale and design. Am Heart J 2007;153(4):478–84.

[36] Mentzer RM Jr, Oz MC, Sladen RN, et al. Effects of perioperative nesiritide in patients with left ventricular dysfunction undergoing cardiac surgery: the NAPA trial. J Am Coll Cardiol 2007;49(6): 716–26.

[37] Sackner-Bernstein JD, Kowalski M, Fox M, et al. Short-term risk of death after treatment with nesiritide for decompensated heart failure: a pooled analysis of randomized controlled trials. JAMA 2005; 293(15):1900–5.

[38] Arora RR, Venkatesh PK, Molnar J. Short and long-term mortality with nesiritide. Am Heart J 2006;152(6):1084–90.

[39] Hauptman PJ, Schnitzler MA, Swindle J, et al. Use of nesiritide before and after publications suggesting drug-related risks in patients with acute decompensated heart failure. JAMA 2006;296(15): 1877–84.

[40] Mitrovic V, Seferovic PM, Simeunovic D, et al. Haemodynamic and clinical effects of ularitide in decompensated heart failure. Eur Heart J 2006;27(23): 2823–32.

[41] Swedberg K, Held P, Kjekshus J, et al. Effects of the early administration of enalapril on mortality in patients with acute myocardial infarction: results of the Cooperative New Scandinavian Enalapril Survival Study II (CONSENSUS II). N Engl J Med 1992; 327(10):678–84.

[42] Cotter G, Kaluski E, Stangl K, et al. The hemodynamic and neurohormonal effects of low doses of tezosentan (an endothelin A/B receptor antagonist) in patients with acute heart failure. Eur J Heart Fail 2004;6(5):601–9.

[43] Torre-Amione G, Young JB, Colucci WS, et al. Hemodynamic and clinical effects of tezosentan, an intravenous dual endothelin receptor antagonist, in patients hospitalized for acute decompensated heart failure. J Am Coll Cardiol 2003;42(1):140–7.

[44] Teerlink JR, Massie BM, Cleland JG, et al. A double-blind, parallel-group, multi-center, placebo-controlled study to investigate the efficacy and safety of tezosentan in reducing symptoms in patients with acute decompensated heart failure [abstract]. Circulation 2001;104:II-526.

[45] McMurray JJV, Teerlink JR, Cotter G, et al. Effects of Tezosentan on Symptoms and Clinical Outcomes in Patients With Acute Heart Failure: The VERITAS Randomized Controlled Trials. JAMA 2007; 298(17):2009–19.

[46] Binkley PF, Starling RC, Hammer DF, et al. Usefulness of hydralazine to withdraw from dobutamine in severe congestive heart failure. Am J Cardiol 1991; 68(10):1103–6.

[47] Bayram M, De Luca L, Massie MB, et al. Reassessment of dobutamine, dopamine, and milrinone in the management of acute heart failure syndromes. Am J Cardiol 2005;96(6A):47G–58G.

[48] Abraham WT, Adams KF, Fonarow GC, et al. In-hospital mortality in patients with acute decompensated heart failure requiring intravenous vasoactive medications: an analysis from the Acute Decompensated Heart Failure National Registry (ADHERE). J Am Coll Cardiol 2005;46(1):57–64.

[49] Elkayam U, Tasissa G, Binanay C, et al. Use and impact of inotropes and vasodilator therapy in hospitalized patients with severe heart failure. Am Heart J 2007;153(1):98–104.

[50] Liang CS, Sherman LG, Doherty JU, et al. Sustained improvement of cardiac function in patients with congestive heart failure after short-term infusion of dobutamine. Circulation 1984; 69(1):113–9.

[51] Burger AJ, Horton DP, LeJemtel T, et al. Effect of nesiritide (B-type natriuretic peptide) and dobutamine on ventricular arrhythmias in the treatment of patients with acutely decompensated congestive heart failure: the PRECEDENT study. Am Heart J 2002;144(6):1102–8.

[52] O'Connor CM, Gattis WA, Uretsky BF, et al. Continuous intravenous dobutamine is associated with an increased risk of death in patients with advanced heart failure: insights from the Flolan International Randomized Survival Trial (FIRST). Am Heart J 1999;138(1 Pt 1):78–86.

[53] Yamani MH, Haji SA, Starling RC, et al. Comparison of dobutamine-based and milrinone-based therapy for advanced decompensated congestive heart failure: hemodynamic efficacy, clinical outcome, and economic impact. Am Heart J 2001;142(6): 998–1002.

[54] Cuffe MS, Califf RM, Adams KF Jr, et al. Short-term intravenous milrinone for acute exacerbation of chronic heart failure: a randomized controlled trial. JAMA 2002;287(12):1541–7.

[55] Felker GM, Benza RL, Chandler AB, et al. Heart failure etiology and response to milrinone in decompensated heart failure: results from the OPTIME-CHF study. J Am Coll Cardiol 2003;41(6):997–1003.

[56] Follath F, Cleland JG, Just H, et al. Efficacy and safety of intravenous levosimendan compared with dobutamine in severe low-output heart failure (the LIDO study): a randomised double-blind trial. Lancet 2002;360(9328):196–202.

[57] Moiseyev VS, Poder P, Andrejevs N, et al. Safety and efficacy of a novel calcium sensitizer, levosimendan, in patients with left ventricular failure due to an acute myocardial infarction: a randomized, placebo-controlled, double-blind study (RUSSLAN). Eur Heart J 2002;23(18):1422–32.

[58] Cleland JG, Ghosh J, Freemantle N, et al. Clinical trials update and cumulative meta-analyses from the American College of Cardiology: WATCH, SCD-HeFT, DINAMIT, CASINO, INSPIRE, STRATUS-US, RIO-Lipids and cardiac resynchronisation therapy in heart failure. Eur J Heart Fail 2004;6(4):501–8.

[59] Packer M, Colucci WS, Fisher L, et al. Development of a comprehensive new endpoint for the evaluation

of new treatments of acute decompensated heart failure: results with levosimendan in the REVIVE-1 study [abstract]. J Card Fail 2003;9:S61.

[60] Cleland JG, Freemantle N, Coletta AP, et al. Clinical trials update from the American Heart Association: REPAIR-AMI, ASTAMI, JELIS, MEGA,

REVIVE-II, SURVIVE, and PROACTIVE. Eur J Heart Fail 2006;8(1):105–10.

[61] Mebazaa A, Nieminen MS, Packer M, et al. Levosimendan vs dobutamine for patients with acute decompensated heart failure: the SURVIVE randomized trial. JAMA 2007;297(17):1883–91.

ELSEVIER
SAUNDERS

Cardiol Clin 25 (2007) 553–564

CARDIOLOGY
CLINICS

Small Pumps for Ventricular Assistance: Progress in Mechanical Circulatory Support

O.H. Frazier, MD*, Leon P. Jacob, MD

Texas Heart Institute at St. Luke's Episcopal Hospital, Houston, TX, USA

In the design of implantable cardiac assist devices, size and durability are critical factors. During the initial clinical experience with left ventricular assist devices (LVADs) for temporary support, success was achieved only with externally placed devices [1]; implantable devices worked from a mechanical standpoint but not from a clinical one [2]. The successful use of long-term implantable LVADs was achieved in the 1980s in bridge-to-transplant patients, using both the HeartMate (Thoratec Corporation, Pleasanton, California) and the Novacor pump (World Heart, Inc., Oakland, California). Clinically, these were outstanding devices for rescuing terminally ill patients with chronic heart failure. Although these pumps saved many lives, it is now clear that pusher-plate technology—with its need for compliance chambers, multiple moving parts, and venting of air pressure—has limitations in terms of pump size, reliability, and durability. The most widely used pulsatile models, the Novacor and HeartMate XVE, have mechanical limitations that necessitate a pump exchange or heart transplant, usually within 18 to 36 months. Furthermore, because pulsatile LVADs are large, many women and other patients with small bodies are excluded from the candidate pool.

To overcome these limitations, cardiologists began in vivo experiments with small, continuous-flow devices in the early 1980s. These efforts culminated in the clinical introduction of the axial-flow Hemopump in 1988 (see below). This simple, efficient technology revolutionized the design of cardiac assist devices, giving rise to a wide range of short- and long-term applications of continous-flow pumps for treating heart failure. Current pumps, based on this principle, are much smaller, simpler, and more efficient. They fit a wider size range of patients and are less invasive to implant. Because they have few moving parts, they are less susceptible to infection and failure. In addition, these pumps offer much greater patient comfort, allowing a relatively normal lifestyle.

This article focuses on the current state of continuous-flow pumps for both temporary and long-term use in treating acute and chronic heart failure.

Continuous-flow pumps for temporary support

Hemopump

The idea of an axial-flow blood pump originated with Dr. Richard Wampler in 1975. While working as a public health consultant in Egypt, he noted that pumps based on the principle of Archimedes' screw (Fig. 1) were being used to supply water to the fields—a practice that had lasted for more than 2000 years. Wampler based the technology used to create the Hemopump on this principle. Clinically, it resulted in a small axial-flow device for temporary, minimally invasive unloading of the failed left ventricle. At a conference in Louisville in 1986, he showed his pump to the senior author, a long-time proponent of continuous flow. Later that year, investigators at the Texas Heart Institute (THI) began laboratory research with the device. The first Hemopump study approved by the United States Food and Drug Administration (FDA) was initiated at THI in April 1988 [3,4].

---

* Corresponding author.

E-mail address: mmallia@heart.thi.tmc.edu
(O.H. Frazier).

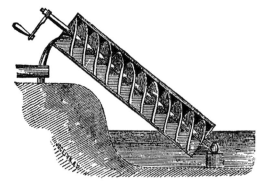

Fig. 1. The principle of Archimedes' screw.

The catheter-mounted pump was inserted through the femoral artery or ascending aorta into the left ventricle. An inlet cannula was placed across the aortic valve, and the pump was positioned above the aortic valve. Components of the Hemopump included the pump assembly, motor unit, and control console. A 20-cm-long radiopaque silicone-rubber inlet cannula, reinforced with a helical spring, was connected to a 7-mm-diameter stainless-steel housing, which surrounded a stainless-steel impeller (Fig. 2). The flexible drive shaft ran from the pump housing to a reusable external motor through a silicone

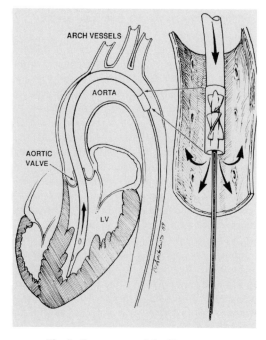

Fig. 2. Components of the Hemopump.

sheath. A purge fluid lubricating system of 50% dextrose supported the rotating element. All the pump surfaces were designed to be blood-contacting. The control console powered the pump, regulated its speed, and calculated the continuous flow.

The principal advantage of the Hemopump was its small size, approximately that of an eraser on a No. 2 lead pencil. The pump speed ranged from 17,000 to 26,000 rpm, generating nonpulsatile flows of 3.5 to 4.5 L/min.

The Hemopump was the first device to reveal the clinical feasibility of using high-speed, implantable rotary pumps for cardiac support [5–8]. Although it yielded a 38% survival rate in a group of more than 150 mortally ill patients, the initial study design was unacceptable to the FDA because of inconsistencies in patient-entry criteria. The FDA asked that the device undergo further evaluation, which the company sponsor was unable to fund. The Hemopump's last owner, the Medtronic Company of Minneapolis, Minnesota, eventually buried the technology in a landfill. Nevertheless, by advancing the options for the treatment of heart failure, the Hemopump paved the way for all subsequent axial-flow LVADs.

Impella

By the early 1990s, the commercial future and widespread application of the Hemopump seemed in doubt. Therefore, the senior author encouraged Helmut Reul at the Helmholtz Institute for Biomedical Engineering in Aachen, Germany, to expand the investigation of Hemopump technology. With the assistance of Thorston Siess, and other researchers at Helmholtz, Reul initiated research that culminated in the Impella Recover System (Impella CardioSystems AG, Aachen, Germany) (Fig. 3). Now undergoing clinical trials, this system, like the Hemopump, is designed to provide immediate, temporary ventricular support in patients whose acute heart failure is not responding to standard medical therapy, as seen in acute myocardial infarctions, life-threatening arrhythmias, or failure to wean from cardiopulmonary bypass. With this device, high-risk coronary bypass has been successfully performed with excellent results.

Three models are available to support the left side of the heart: the Recover LD 5.0 (surgically implanted directly into the left ventricle), the Recover LP 5.0 LVAD (advanced into the left ventricle via an arterial cutdown in the groin), and

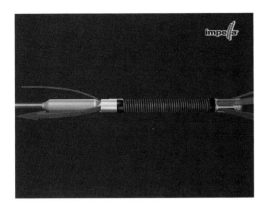

Fig. 3. Impella Recover LP 5.0 Left Ventricular Assist Device.

the Recover LP 2.5 (inserted percutaneously). Another model, the Recover RD, is employed for right ventricular support [9]. Because the Impella Recover System may be used in both sides of the heart, its technology is unique among small pumps.

The pump, including the cannula, measures 6.0 cm in length, 4.0 mm in diameter (12F) for the percutaneous device, and 6.4 mm in diameter for the surgically implanted device. The Recover LD and LP 5.0 models can provide continuous flows of up to 4.5 L/min at 33,000 rpm for as long as 7 days. The LP 5.0 catheter size ranges from 9F at the distal end, where the pump is located, to 21F at the proximal end, which contains the pump housing. The catheter shaft contains the electrical connections for the pump motor sensor and a separate tube for transferring fluid via a purge system. The percutaneous Recover LP 2.5 delivers 2.5 L/min of blood and can provide support for up to 5 days.

Clinical experience was initiated in 2003 by Meyns and colleagues [10], in Belgium, with operative insertion of the LD 5.0 model in patients with cardiogenic shock. Further clinical experience in Europe has shown the device to be highly effective for unloading the acutely failed left ventricle with minimal device-related complications [11]. It can safely improve end-organ perfusion, cardiac output, and other hemodynamic parameters in patients with cardiac shock [12–18].

Currently, the Impella Recover System has been used in more than 1000 patients in Europe. In the United States, AbioMed, of Danvers, Massachusetts, the current owner of this technology, has initiated clinical trials of both the percutaneous LP

2.5 and the larger (LP 5.0) device. For both cardiologists and cardiac surgeons, the Impella offers hope for providing a simple, effective means of temporarily unloading the left ventricle.

TandemHeart

The use of an external pump to provide temporary cardiac support by means of a non-surgical approach is not a new concept. In 1962, Dennis and colleagues [19,20] reported their experience with this approach in treating eight patients with acute cardiogenic shock related to myocardial infarction. The left atrial inlet cannula was placed in the internal jugular vein by means of simple tactile location of the fossa ovalis. After transseptal perforation was performed, the left atrium was unloaded directly by an external roller pump, and blood was returned via the femoral artery. Because revascularization therapies were not yet available, none of Dennis's patients survived long-term. Nevertheless, the concept was successfully applied in seven of the eight patients.

More recently, the advent of the TandemHeart percutaneous ventricular assist device (CardiacAssist, Inc., Pittsburgh, Pennsylvania) (Fig. 4), has resulted in the clinically meaningful application of that earlier concept [21–24]. The TandemHeart, which began to be developed in 1991, weighs 227 g and operates at 3000 to 7500 rpm, supplying up to 4 L/min of continuous cardiac output [25]. In 2002, the FDA granted 17 sites approval to study the device [26]. Designed for temporary use, this continuous-flow LVAD may be appropriate in several clinical settings, especially those involving cardiac shock. Although the TandemHeart can be inserted by cardiovascular surgeons in the operating room, its most usual and effective application is by cardiologists in the catheterization laboratory.

In either setting, a transatrial-septal cannula is advanced into the left atrium (from the right atrium). Inflow is achieved with a 21F cannula placed in the left atrium through an atrial transseptal puncture via the femoral vein. A 15F to 17F femoral artery outflow cannula is placed in the femoral artery. The cannula draws oxygenated blood from the left atrium into an external centrifugal pump. This dual-chambered pump has both an upper and a lower housing. Blood flows through the upper housing, and the lower housing provides the power assembly. The latter includes a communicating link to the controller, which rotates the impeller, as well as an anticoagulant

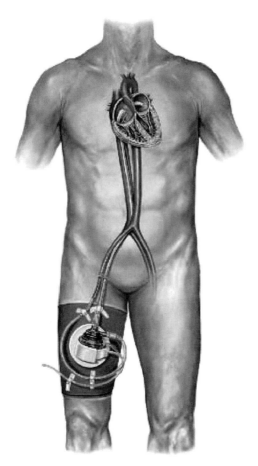

Fig. 4. TandemHeart Percutaneous Ventricular Assist Device. (*Reprinted from* La Francesca S, Palanichamy N, Kar B, et al. First use of the TandemHeart percutaneous left ventricular assist device as a short-term bridge to cardiac transplantation. Tex Heart Inst J. 2006;33(4):491.)

infusion line, which protects the hydrodynamic bearing by cooling and anticoagulating it.

Clinical use of the TandemHeart has been encouraging, with documented percutaneous reversal of cardiogenic shock, as first reported by Thiele and associates [27], improved survival at both THI and other centers. We have recently documented excellent survival rates in patients with severe refractory cardiogenic shock [28]. We have also used the TandemHeart as an adjunct to high-risk surgery [26]. In 34 additional surgical patients, we have used this device as a bridge to either transplantation, high-risk valvular and revascularization surgery, or long-term LVAD use. Support periods have ranged from a few hours to 1 month in duration.

Continuous-flow pumps for long-term support

Jarvik Heart

In 1989, we began initial developement of a long-term, implantable pump with nonlubricated bearings (the Jarvik 2000 Heart; Jarvik Heart, Inc., New York, New York) in collaboration with Dr. Robert Jarvik. Extensive animal tests verified the feasibility of using implantable nonlubricated bearings. By 1994, complication-free support periods of up to 10 months had been achieved. Because of this pump's small size and the inherent complications of the inflow cannula in other technologies, the senior author recommended intraventricular implantation [29,30], and this has indeed been the approach used. The first clinical implant occurred in 1999 [31], and the initial clinical bridge-to-transplant trial began in April 2000. Two months later, a destination-therapy trial was initiated with Stephen Westaby in Oxford, England.

The current blood pump (Fig. 5) is made of titanium and about the size of a common C-cell battery. It weighs 90 g, measures 2.5 cm in diameter, and displaces 25 mL. Within the pump housing is a sealed, brushless, electromagnetic, direct-current motor. The rotor is held in place by two ceramic bearings. The device can pump up to 7 L/min against physiologic resistance. The recent addition of sintered titanium microspheres on its intraventricular blood-contacting

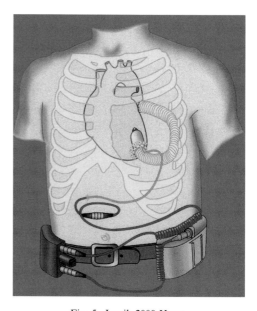

Fig. 5. Jarvik 2000 Heart.

surfaces, as well as a phased controller that lowers the pump speed to 7000 rpm for 6 seconds every minute, has lessened the most common clinical complications associated with the use of this pump. These complications include thrombus around the base of the pump in the ventricle (addressed by the sintered titanium microspheres), thrombus in the noncoronary aortic cusp when aortic valve opening is limited or absent (addressed by the intermittent speed controller), and a septal shift impairing right ventricular function (addressed by the intermittent speed controller). The pump is powered by lithium ion batteries, each of which lasts up to 8 hours. Power is transmitted by means of insulated cables enclosed within a silicone tube. The power cable is commonly brought out through the right subcostal margin, but an alternative skull-pedestal power-cable connector has been used in Europe for destination-therapy patients (Fig. 6) [32].

The Jarvik Heart is also unique in that it has an external speed control that can easily be changed by the patient or physician according to physiologic needs. The speed control allows variations from 8000 to 12,000 rpm. This pump has the longest in vivo durability, with over 7 years of continuous support in a destination-therapy patient who received it in June 2000 in Oxford [33]. The pump is connected to the arterial circulation by a 16-mm Hemashield outflow graft. Initially, this graft was placed in the descending thoracic aorta, but other sites have been used successfully, including the supraceliac aorta, the ascending aorta, and the first part of the descending aorta [34]. In most cases, the pump can be placed without cardiopulmonary bypass [35]. This enhances its usefulness in critically ill patients with chronic heart failure. Placement through a subcostal incision may be of value in redo sternotomy patients (Fig. 7) [36].

This technology has had minimal infectious complications, and there have been no pump failures due to mechanical bearing wear or pump thrombosis. A failure mode has not been

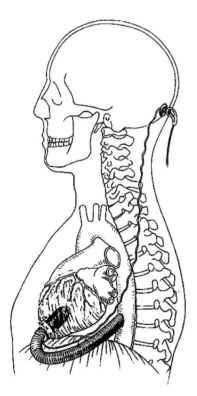

Fig. 6. An alternative version of the Jarvik 2000 system incorporates a titanium pedestal mounted to the posterior portion of the skull. The power and control connection is made just outside the skin. (*Reprinted from* Westaby S, Katsumata T, Evan R, et al. The Jarvik 2000 oxford system: increasing the scope of mechanical circulatory support. J Thorac Cardiovasc Surg 1997;114:469; with permission.)

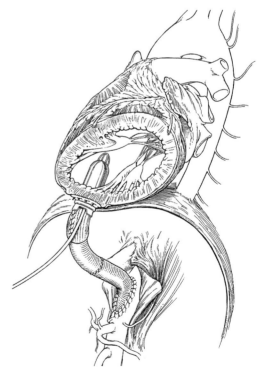

Fig. 7. Jarvik 2000: subcostal placement.

demonstrated, either in vitro or in vivo [37]. Optimal clinical use is achieved when the Jarvik 2000 works in parallel with the native heart, ie, when the native ventricle is ejecting and the Jarvik pump unloading the ventricle throughout the cardiac cycle (Fig. 8) [38]. In general, early mortality has been related to an excessive septal shift that compromises right ventricular function and to thrombus formation in the aortic root and ventricular cavity. Modifications of this pump and a better understanding of the altered physiology that it induces should alleviate these problems in the future.

According to the manufacturer, as of August 2007, the Jarvik 2000 pump had been placed in more than 219 patients at 35 centers in Europe and elsewhere. It is now undergoing a bridge-to-transplant trial in the United States and has received the CE mark in Europe for both destination therapy and bridging to transplantation.

HeartMate II

Initial development of the HeartMate II began during the early Hemopump trials. As medical advisor to the Nimbus Corporation (Rancho

Cordova, California), the senior author suggested that, instead of pursuing a magnetically suspended axial-flow pump, the company should merely add implantable bearings to the Hemopump and make it larger and more durable for long-term support. Further development of this technology was advanced by the Nimbus company at the University of Pittsburgh's McGowan Center. The device was refined for clinical use by the Thoratec Corporation, which acquired this technology in 2000.

The HeartMate II is an implantable axial-flow system comprising a small pump, controller module, power base unit, and portable battery (Fig. 9). The impeller, the pump's only moving part, spins on blood-lubricated bearings powered by an electromagnetic motor. The blood-contacting inflow cannula is coated with sintered titanium. The single driveline is brought out through the right side of the abdomen and connected to the controller, which operates the motor.

At 4 cm in diameter, 6 cm in length, and 375 g in weight, the pump units are considerably smaller than those of the HeartMate I. Speeds range from 6000 to 15,000 rpm, offering up to 10.0 L/min of continuous output. Like other continuous-flow

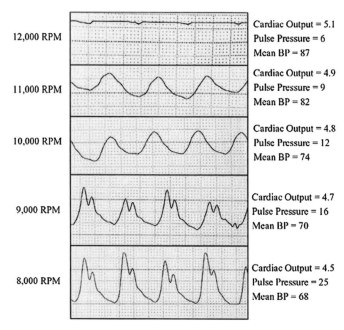

Fig. 8. Jarvik 2000: arterial pressure tracing at standard pump speed settings. At 8000 and 9000 rpm the aortic valve is opening, whereas above 10,000 rpm the aortic valve remains closed. The pulse pressure decreases from 25 mm Hg at 8000 rpm to 6 mm Hg at 12,000 rpm. (BP = blood pressure.) (*Reprinted from* Frazier OH, Myers TJ, Gregoric ID, et al. Initial clinical experience with the Jarvik 2000 implantable axial-flow left ventricular assist system. Circulation 2002;105(24):2858; with permission.)

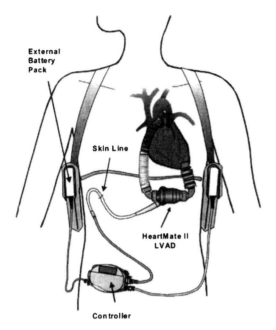

Fig. 9. HeartMate II Left Ventricular Assist Device.

pumps, this device has the potential for an automated speed mode. Owing to the unreliability of this technology, however, the pump is being operated only as a fixed-speed device, the suitable speed being determined at the time of implantation.

In Europe, clinical trials of the HeartMate II began in 2000. The initial experience was unfavorable, particularly because of thrombus formation near the inflow and outflow stators, close to the fore and aft bearings [39]. Researchers redesigned the pump by removing the textured surfaces on the stators and replacing them with smooth surfaces.

In the United States, the first redesigned HeartMate II implant was performed at THI in November 2003 in an 18-year-old boy with dilated cardiomyopathy [26]. The following year, the FDA granted this patient permission to return home while awaiting a transplant. So far, the HeartMate II has been used primarily as a bridge-to-transplant therapy, but researchers have recently begun to study it as a bridge to recovery. As of August 2007, five HeartMate II recipients whose devices were implanted for chronic congestive heart failure (not myocarditis) have successfully had their pumps removed. Four of these patients were slowly weaned from pump support after undergoing successful cardiac

rehabilitation. The fifth patient underwent device removal due to a driveline malfunction and now has acceptable cardiac function with medical therapy. Such patients are considered to be in remission from congestive heart failure rather than recovered, as their disease is of unknown etiology and duration. Until further long-term data are accumulated in such cases, afterload-reduction therapy will continue to be maintained.

The recently published results of the initial multicenter clinical trial, performed at 26 centers, were favorable. Experiences with the devices varied widely in these centers, many of which had had minimal involvement with LVAD technology prior to this study. Despite the expected operative mishaps, errors in patient selection, and errors in pump assembly, 100 (75%) of the 133 patients had successful outcomes, meeting the principal endpoint of undergoing transplantation or being successfully supported for 180 days on the active transplant list [40]. There were no technology-related failures, although one patient had a broken inflow cable after falling off his skateboard. He survived the pump exchange [41] and, indeed, is a tribute to the functional recovery level achievable with pump support alone.

The HeartMate II is the first device to be manufactured and marketed by a company that does not depend primarily on research for its operational activities. Because of the pump's reliability and minimal infectious complications, it should be considered more than simply a rescue device. Indeed, it should be safely used in New York Heart Association functional Class III patients or homebound Class IV patients. By expanding treatment options, the HeartMate II has paved the way for wider application of continuous-flow blood pump technology and its meaningful clinical benefits.

MicroMed DeBakey LVAD

The MicroMed DeBakey LVAD (Fig. 10) (MicroMed Cardiovascular, Inc., Houston, Texas) is the first long-term, implantable, axial-flow pump to have been used clinically. The system comprises a pump, a controller module, battery packs, a battery charger, and a home support system or clinical data acquisition system. The pump measures 86 mm by 25 mm and weighs only 95 g. Inside the titanium pump housing, the inducer-impeller is the only moving part. The pump is attached to a curved titanium inflow cannula and a Dacron outflow graft that is surrounded by a permanent

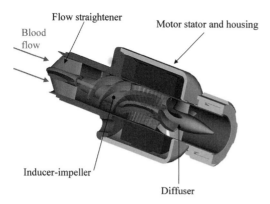

Fig. 10. MicroMed DeBakey Left Ventricular Assist Device.

ultrasonic flow probe. A single driveline cable is tunneled through the abdomen and connected to the external control module. The pump operates at 7500 to 12,500 rpm and can provide more than 10.0 L/min of continuous cardiac output [42].

The MicroMed DeBakey pump was first implanted in November 1998 in Berlin and has been widely used since that time. The worldwide experience reported by Goldstein [43] involved 150 patients at 14 centers over a 3.5-year period. Although the experience was favorable, pump thrombus was noted in 11% of the patients and thromboembolic events in 10%. Though no relationship was noted between the neurologic events and pump thrombus, the manufacturer redesigned

the pump bearings and added a special synthetic coating called Carmeda to the pump. Unfortunately, the Carmeda-coated pump was also fraught with pump thrombus problems, leading to two more iterations of this technology. The fourth iteration seems favorable, although only a small number of patients have received it. The pump's advantages include its small size and its ability to be implanted, in most cases, totally within the thoracic cavity. The pump also seems to provide the most accurate recording of pump output of any device in current clinical use.

Magnetically suspended centrifugal pumps

Because the initial axial-flow pumps had mechanical bearings which could potentially become worn, researchers began to develop implantable, magnetically suspended pumps, which have the potential for longer durability. Most of these pumps have a magnetically levitated (maglev) impeller that eliminates the need for mechanical bearings and physical contact between moving parts. By generating higher torque at a lower speed, these pumps should minimize wear, heat generation, and hemolysis. Several maglev designs are being developed and should soon see widespread use.

DuraHeart

Research on the implantable DuraHeart (Terumo Heart, Inc., Ann Arbor, Michigan) (Fig. 11),

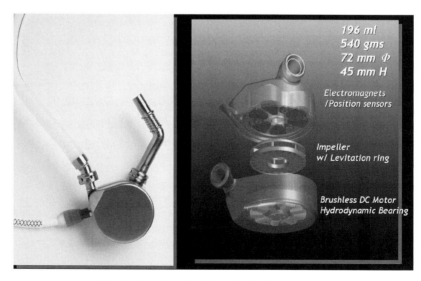

Fig. 11. DuraHeart Left Ventricular Assist System.

has been ongoing since 1995 [44]. The external casing of this implantable centrifugal assist device contains a maglev impeller. On each side of the impeller is a magnet, which exerts a rotational force on the impeller. Opposite the impeller is a ferromagnetic ring that stabilizes the electromagnetic sphere. A sensor unit distributes the electromagnetic forces to ensure that the impeller remains centered within the blood chamber. In addition, the lower part of the pump housing contains a hydrodynamic bearing for use in case of magnetic-bearing failure. The inflow and outflow ports are perpendicular to the pump housing, the inflow entering the proximal pump housing and the outflow being tangential to the impeller path. The pump unit weighs 540 g, measures 72 by 45 mm, and has a displacement volume of 180 cm^3. External components include a controller and battery pack, which is connected to the pump through a percutaneous driveline tunneled through the abdomen. Operating at 1200 to 2600 rpm, the DuraHeart yields 2 to 10 L/min of continuous flow [45]. The lack of mechanical contact should theoretically enhance the pump's durability and reliability.

The DuraHeart was first implanted clinically in early 2004 at the Ruhr University of Bochum [46]. As of February 2007, it had been used in 33 patients, for a cumulative support duration of more than 5000 days. Twelve patients were supported for more than 6 months and four patients for more than 12 months (including one patient for more than 600 days). Seventy-nine percent of the patients met the primary endpoint of transplantation or survival at 13 weeks [47,48].

Although further experience is necessary to clarify the role of the DuraHeart, it is already showing considerable promise in the treatment of congestive heart failure.

Levitronix CentriMag

The Levitronix CentriMag (Thoratec Corporation) (Fig. 12) is a maglev pump in which an impeller operates in a bearingless, or "self-bearing," rotor that floats with a rotating magnetic field. This rotor is suspended by eight L-shaped iron cores that create a contact-free environment. Operating in the relatively low range of 1500 to 5500 rpm, the pump delivers up to 9.9 L/min of continuous flow [49]. Whereas the inlet is on the same rotational axis as the rotor, the outlet is perpendicular to the inlet and oriented tangentially to the pump. Because of its contact-free environment

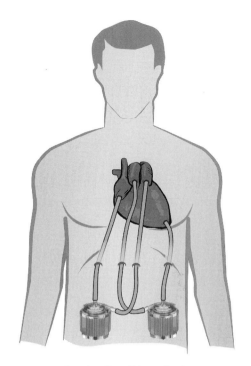

Fig. 12. Levitronix CentriMag circulatory support pump.

and absence of seals or valves, this device minimizes blood trauma, virtually eliminating hemolysis and thrombus formation.

Clinical trials of the CentriMag began in 2003. It is currently being marketed as a quickly implantable device for short-term use in patients with potentially recoverable heart failure. It has proved valuable for stabilizing patients with multiorgan system failure and an uncertain neurologic status [50]. By placing the cannula through a graft [50,51], THI has used this method in the past to avoid reopening the chest when weaning is deemed adequate. In this case, the inlet cannula is removed from the inside of the graft, and the graft is oversewn. The outflow graft may be similarly oversewn. The CentriMag pump is widely used for short-term cardiac support in both Europe and the United States.

INCOR

The INCOR (Berlin Heart GmbH, Berlin, Germany) (Fig. 13), the first magnetically suspended, axial-flow pump to undergo clinical application, was initially implanted in 2002 at the German Heart Institute, in Berlin. Within the pump's titanium housing, the blood-contacting

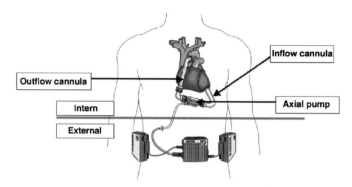

Fig. 13. INCOR Left Ventricular Assist Device. (*Reprinted from* Huber CH, Tozzi P, Humi M, et al. No drive line, no seal, no bearing and no wear: magnetics for impeller suspension and flow assessment in a new VAD. Interact Cardiovasc Thorac Surg 2004;3:337; with permission.)

surfaces are heparin coated. The silicone inflow cannula is inserted into the left ventricular apex, and the adjustable-length silicone outflow cannula is anastomosed to the ascending aorta. Axial levitation is achieved with electromagnets mounted at both ends of the impeller. The rotor position is controlled by a sensor system that creates constant laminar flow, thus avoiding mechanical wear [52].

The pump is powered via a driveline that exits from the right side of the abdomen and is connected to a controller and two battery packs. It weighs 200 g and measures 30 mm by 12 cm. Operating at 5000 to 10,000 rpm, it can provide up to 7 L/min of continuous outflow [53].

By the end of 2006, 212 INCOR pumps had been implanted worldwide. Although currently being used as a bridge to recovery or transplantation, the INCOR was designed specifically for long-term destination therapy. Further studies are

needed, both clinically and experimentally, to clarify this device's role in supporting the heart.

HeartWare

The HeartWare [54] (Fig. 14) is a small, continuous-flow, centrifugal pump that uses a hybrid system (a combination of passive magnets and a hydrodynamic thruster) for suspending the impeller, the only moving part within the pump. The hydrodynamic thruster's bearing establishes a cushion of blood between the impeller and the pump housing. Once power is applied to the device, there are no points of mechanical contact within the pump. This feature is expected to improve device reliability and reduce the risk of blood trauma as cells pass through the pump. The HeartWare can generate up to 10 L/min of forward flow and can be implanted within the pericardial sac, avoiding abdominal surgery. It is undergoing limited trials in Europe.

Summary

Today's small pumps have greatly expanded the options for treating both acute and chronic heart failure. Unexpectedly, continuous-flow pumps with bearings have evidenced minimal device wear. The longest support period is now more than 7 years in a Jarvik Heart recipient, and the pump shows no evidence of bearing wear. Similar results have been observed with the HeartMate II pump. The lack of infection, ease of implantability, and ease of explantability are additional reasons to consider using these pumps before patients enter the terminal stages of heart failure. Early interruption of the heart failure cascade may lead to a higher incidence of

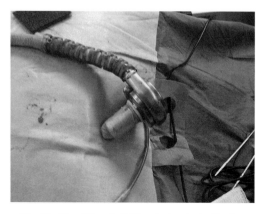

Fig. 14. HeartWare Left Ventricular Assist Device.

remission of heart failure and ultimate device removal. Ongoing technological advances will give rise to even better device-related therapies in the future.

References

[1] Ross JN Jr, Wieting DW, Hall CW, et al. Use of a paracorporeal left ventricular bypass pump in experimental heart failure. Am J Cardiol 1971;27:12–9.
[2] Norman JC. ALVAD 1979: precedence, potentials, prospects and problems. Cardiovasc Dis 1979;6: 384–9.
[3] Frazier OH, Wampler RK, Duncan JM, et al. First human use of the Hemopump, a catheter-mounted ventricular assist device. Ann Thorac Surg 1990;49: 299–304.
[4] Wampler RK, Moise JC, Frazier OH, et al. *In vivo* evaluation of a peripheral vascular access axial flow blood pump. Trans Am Soc Artif Intern Organs 1988;34:450–4.
[5] Meyns B, Nishimura Y, Racz R, et al. Organ perfusion with Hemopump device assistance with and without intraaortic balloon pumping. J Thorac Cardiovasc Surg 1997;114:243–53.
[6] Scholz KH, Dubois-Rande JL, Urban P, et al. Clinical experience with the percutaneous hemopump during high-risk coronary angioplasty. Am J Cardiol 1998;82:1107–10.
[7] Sweeney MS. The Hemopump in 1997: a clinical, political, and marketing evolution. Ann Thorac Surg 1999;68:761–3.
[8] Meyns B, Sergeant P, Wouters P, et al. Mechanical support with microaxial blood pumps for postcardiotomy left ventricular failure: can outcome be predicted? J Thorac Cardiovasc Surg 2000;120:393–400.
[9] Brinton TJ, Fitzgerald PJ. Ventricular assist technologies. In: Tremmel J, editor. SIS 2006 yearbook. Seattle (WA): Science Innovation Synergy; 2006. p. 159–68.
[10] Meyns B, Dens J, Sergeant P, et al. Initial experiences with the Impella device in patients with cardiogenic shock: Impella support for cardiogenic shock. Thorac Cardiovasc Surg 2003;51:312–7.
[11] Jurmann MJ, Siniawski H, Erb M, et al. Initial experience with miniature axial flow ventricular assist devices for postcardiotomy heart failure. Ann Thorac Surg 2004;77:1642–7.
[12] Colombo T, Garatti A, Bruschi G, et al. First successful bridge to recovery with the Impella Recover 100 left ventricular assist device for fulminant acute myocarditis. Ital Heart J 2003;4:642–5.
[13] Siegenthaler MP, Brehm K, Strecker T, et al. The Impella Recover microaxial left ventricular assist device reduces mortality for postcardiotomy failure: a three-center experience. J Thorac Cardiovasc Surg 2004;127:812–22.
[14] Garatti A, Colombo T, Russo C, et al. Different applications for the left ventricular mechanical support with the impella recover 100 microaxial blood pump. J Heart Lung Transplant 2004;24:481–5.
[15] Meyns B, Autschbach R, Boning A, et al. Coronary artery bypass grafting supported with intracardiac microaxial pumps versus normothermic cardiopulmonary bypass: a prospective randomised trial. Eur J Cardiothorac Surg 2002;22:112–7.
[16] Meyns B, Stolinski J, Leunens V, et al. Left ventricular support by catheter-mounted axial flow pump reduces infarct size. J Am Coll Cardiol 2003;41: 1087–95.
[17] Kaufmann R, Rakhorst G, Mihaylov D, et al. A novel implantable electromechanical ventricular assist device. First acute animal testing. ASAIO J 1997;43:360–2.
[18] Forster F, Kaufmann R, Reul H, et al. A small pulsatile blood pump for ventricular support during end-stage heart failure. Artif Organs 2000;24:373–6.
[19] Dennis C, Carlens C, Senning A, et al. Clinical use of a cannula for left heart bypass without thoracotomy. Ann Surg 1962;156:623–37.
[20] Ross JJ, Braunwald E, Morrow A. Left heart catheterization by the transseptal route: a description of the technique and complications. Circulation 1960; 22:927–34.
[21] Satoh H, Kobayashi T, Nakano S, et al. Clinical application of percutaneous left ventricular support with a centrifugal pump. ASAIO J 1993;39:153–5.
[22] Edmunds LH Jr, Herrmann HC, DiSesa VJ, et al. Left ventricular assist without thoracotomy: clinical experience with the Dennis method. Ann Thorac Surg 1994;57:880–5.
[23] Fonger JD, Zhou Y, Matsuura H, et al. Enhanced preservation of acutely ischemic myocardium with transseptal left ventricular assist. Ann Thorac Surg 1994;57:570–5.
[24] Pavie A, Leger P, Nzomvuama A, et al. Left centrifugal pump cardiac assist with transseptal percutaneous left atrial cannula. Artif Organs 1998;22:502–7.
[25] Kar B, Adkins LE, Civitello AB, et al. Clinical experience with the tandemheart percutaneous ventricular assist device. Tex Heart Inst J 2006;33:111–5.
[26] Gemmato CJ, Forrester MD, Myers TJ, et al. Thirty-five years of mechanical circulatory support at the Texas Heart Institute: an updated overview. Tex Heart Inst J 2005;32:168–77.
[27] Thiele H, Lauer B, Hambrecht R, et al. Reversal of cardiogenic shock by percutaneous left atrial-to-femoral arterial bypass assistance. Circulation 2001;104:2917–22.
[28] Idelchik GM, Loyalka P, Kar B. Percutaneous ventricular assist device placement during active cardiopulmonary resuscitation for severe refractory cardiogenic shock after acute myocardial infarction. Tex Heart Inst J 2007;34:204–8.
[29] Frank CM, Palanichamy N, Kar B, et al. Use of a percutaneous ventricular assist device for

treatment of cardiogenic shock due to critical aortic stenosis. Tex Heart Inst J 2006;33:487–9.

[30] Frazier OH, Myers TJ, Westaby S, et al. Use of the Jarvik 2000 left ventricular assist system as a bridge to heart transplantation or as destination therapy for patients with chronic heart failure. Ann Surg 2003; 237:631–7.

[31] Cooley DA. Initial clinical experience with the Jarvik 2000 implantable axial-flow left ventricular assist system. Circulation 2002;105:2808–9.

[32] Frazier OH, Myers TJ, Jarvik RK, et al. Research and development of an implantable, axial-flow left ventricular assist device: the Jarvik 2000 Heart. Ann Thorac Surg 2001;71:S125–32.

[33] Westaby S, Frazier OH, Banning A. Six years of continuous mechanical circulatory support. N Engl J Med 2006;355:325–7.

[34] Myers T, Frazier OH, Delgado R. Use of mechanical devices in treating heart failure. In: Hosenpud J, Greenberg B, editors. Congestive heart failure. 3rd edition. Philadelphia: Lippincott Williams & Wilkins; 2006. p. 776–81.

[35] Frazier OH. Implantation of the Jarvik 2000 left ventricular assist device without the use of cardiopulmonary bypass. Ann Thorac Surg 2003;75: 1028–30.

[36] Westaby S, Frazier OH, Pigott DW, et al. Implant technique for the Jarvik 2000 Heart. Ann Thorac Surg 2002;73:1337–40.

[37] Siegenthaler MP, Frazier OH, Beyersdorf F, et al. Mechanical reliability of the Jarvik 2000 heart. Ann Thorac Surg 2006;81:1752–8.

[38] Frazier OH, Myers TJ, Westaby S, et al. Clinical experience with an implantable, intracardiac, continuous flow circulatory support device: physiologic implications and their relationship to patient selection. Ann Thorac Surg 2004;77:133–42.

[39] Frazier OH, Delgado RM III, Kar B, et al. First clinical use of the redesigned HeartMate II left ventricular assist system in the United States: a case report. Tex Heart Inst J 2004;31:157–9.

[40] Miller LW, Pagani FD, Russell SD, et al. Use of a continuous-flow device in patients awaiting heart transplantation. N Engl J Med 2007;357:885–96.

[41] La Francesca S, Smith R, Gregoric ID, et al. Replacement of a malfunctioning HeartMate II left ventricular assist device in a 14-year-old after a sudden fall. J Heart Lung Transplant 2006;25(7):862–4.

[42] DeBakey ME, Teitel ER. Use of the MicroMed DeBakey VAD for the treatment of end-stage heart failure. Expert Rev Med Devices 2005;2:137–40.

[43] Goldstein DJ. Worldwide experienced with the MicroMed DeBakey ventricular assist device® as a bridge to transplantation. Circulation 2003;108: II-272–7.

[44] Akamatsu T, Tsukiya T, Nishimura K, et al. Recent studies of the centrifugal blood pump with a magnetically suspended impeller. Artif Organs 1995;19: 631–4.

[45] Komoda T, Weng Y, Nojiri C, et al. Implantation technique for the DuraHeart left ventricular assist system. J Artif Organs 2007;10:124–7.

[46] Terumo Heart, Inc. Announces the first implant of the DuraHeart left left ventricular assist system. Available at: http://www.terumo-cvs.com/news_and_events/render_news.asp?newsId=5. Accessed August 24, 2007.

[47] Terumo Heart, Inc. Press release. Available at: http://www.terumoheart.com/news_pr.asp. Accessed August 24, 2007.

[48] El-Banayosy A, Koerfer R, Hetzer R, et al. Initial results of a European multicenter clinical trial with the DuraHeart Mag-Lev centrifugal left ventricular assist device. J Heart Lung Transplant 2006;25:145.

[49] Texas Heart Institute. Heart assist devices: Levitronix CentriMag LVAS. Available at: http://www.texasheartinstitute.org/Research/Devices/levitronix.cfm. Accessed August 24, 2007.

[50] John R, Liao K, Lietz K, et al. Experience with the Levitronix CentriMag circulatory support system as a bridge to decision in patients with refractory acute cardiogenic shock and multisystem organ failure. J Thorac Cardiovasc Surg 2007;134: 351–8.

[51] De Robertis F, Birks EJ, Rogers P, et al. Clinical performance with the levitronix centrimag short-term ventricular assist device. J Heart Lung Transplant 2006;25:181–6 [Epub 2006 Jan 6].

[52] Berlin Heart website. Available at: http://www.berlinheart.de. Accessed August 24, 2007.

[53] Huber CH, Tozzi P, Hurni M, et al. No drive line, no seal, no bearing and no wear: magnetics for impeller suspension and flow assessment in a new VAD. Interact Cardiovasc Thorac Surg 2004;3:336–40.

[54] Available at: http://www.heartware.com.au/IRM/content/usa/home.html. Accessed August 31, 2007.

ELSEVIER
SAUNDERS

Cardiol Clin 25 (2007) 565–571

Invasive Hemodynamic Monitoring the Aftermath of the ESCAPE Trial

Carl V. Leier, MD

The Ohio State University, Columbus, OH, USA

This article specifically addresses the use of right-sided heart catheterization with a balloon-tip, flow-directed, indwelling pulmonary artery catheter (ie, Swan-Ganz catheter) in managing the heart failure patient. Indwelling arterial conduits and the newer still experimental devices for long-term monitoring and recording of pressures (eg, pulmonary artery, left atrial) or impedance are not discussed herein.

Instrumentation and devices of all sorts have a major role in the diagnosis and management of cardiovascular disease. The Swan-Ganz pulmonary artery catheter (PAC), one such device, has a storied past; however, the results of several trials indicate that the PAC will have a more restrained future.

The journey and heyday

The placement of a catheter within cardiac chambers via the venous system was first published by Forssmann [1] in 1929. Using ureteral catheters ("4 charrieres thickness"), he developed a cardiac catheterization technique on human cadavers and confirmed positioning of the catheters at autopsy. With the assistance of a surgical colleague, Forssmann placed the first cardiac catheter ("well oiled") in a living human in himself via an "elbow vein," and after walking "a long way from the operating room to the x-ray room," he radiographically confirmed termination of the catheter in the right atrium. The primary objective of his work was to develop a method for proficient and reliable delivery of medications to the heart and a more rapid systemic distribution while avoiding the immensely high risk of transthoracic intracardiac injections and infusions.

Cournand and Ranges [2] and Cournand and colleagues [3] respectively reported the use of right-sided heart catheterization as a means of accurately measuring cardiac output (1941) and right heart pressures (1944). In 1949, Hellems and colleagues [4] from the laboratory of Louis Dexter reported the concept and use of pulmonary "capillary" pressure in humans, which was correlated with left atrial pressure by Connolly and colleagues [5] in 1954. Thereafter, right-sided heart catheterization became the standard invasive cardiac diagnostic study, joined by left-sided heart catheterization over the ensuing decade.

The impact article on the use of PACs in human cardiac failure was published in 1970 [6]. This report linked the name "Swan-Ganz" for the primary researchers and lead investigators, H.J.C. Swan and W. Ganz, to the catheter specifically designed for continuous monitoring of right-sided heart and pulmonary artery pressures, and with inflation of the balloon located near the catheter tip, intermittent pulmonary artery occlusive ("capillary wedge") pressure. The operator-controlled, balloon-tip afforded relatively easy and rapid flotation positioning, allowing placement at the bedside without the need for radiography in most patients. A thermistor near the catheter tip added the thermodilution method for cardiac output determinations using temperature as the volume-flow indicator [7]. Over the ensuing 30 years, other options (eg, pacing electrodes, additional lumens) were added to serve various investigative and clinical needs.

The heyday of the Swan-Ganz PAC occurred in the last quarter of the twentieth century. The PAC allowed direct and continuous measurement

E-mail address: carl.leier@osumc.edu

of central hemodynamic parameters for several days after insertion. Sequential recordings could be made in various body positions, during exercise and other perturbations, and following interventions. Drug development (and approval for clinical application) in heart failure during this era invariably required a hemodynamic profile rendered by the PAC of each agent under study. Preload-reducing agents were primarily characterized by their ability to decrease ventricular diastolic filling pressures, estimated by right atrial and pulmonary artery occlusive pressures. Afterload-reducing agents primarily caused a reduction in calculated vascular resistance with a consequent rise in stroke volume and cardiac output. Positive inotropic drugs had to demonstrate the ability to primarily augment cardiac contractility, stroke volume, and cardiac output with varying vascular effects depending on the agent tested. These hemodynamic properties were characterized for each agent under study during this era via data obtained from the Swan-Ganz PAC.

In the 1990s, the winds began to change from routine use of the PAC in drug development, evaluation, and approval for heart failure to other generally less invasive approaches. This shift occurred when it was learned that the initial or short-term hemodynamic profile of a drug, even if favorable, did not predict its long-term hemodynamic effects or clinical outcomes when the drug was repeatedly administered over time [8–11]. Drug evaluation in heart failure appropriately moved to simple or optional hemodynamic characterization with an overwhelming emphasis placed on clinical outcomes, symptom relief, activity (physical) tolerance, survival, and, more recently, effects on cardiac or vascular remodeling.

Nevertheless, the PAC remains an important investigative device in the development of drugs and interventions for managing acute heart failure. The hemodynamic profile of an agent must be reasonably well defined and characterized before its approval and widespread use in this urgent, typically tenuous clinical situation. In contrast, the role of the PAC is now more restrained in the investigation of interventions for decompensated chronic heart failure, which is often erroneously placed under the category of acute heart failure.

The non-research oriented, general clinical application of the PAC has followed a similar course, perhaps with a 10-year hysteresis, from widespread use to a waning role. Much of the withdrawal from widespread use of the PAC in clinical medicine was prompted by the results of several retrospective studies and prospective trials specifically addressing the merits of routine use of the PAC in the management of heart failure and other critical care conditions.

Studies and trials addressing the use of the pulmonary arterial catheter

Although the PAC was used extensively to evaluate innumerable pharmacologic agents in heart failure and to investigate, evaluate, and manage other serious clinical conditions (eg, septic shock, adult respiratory distress), the use of the PAC itself did not undergo any noteworthy scrutiny during its first 10 to 15 years of employment as an investigative or clinical device. Although small or retrospective studies appeared to justify the use of the PAC to improve outcomes in various clinical conditions [12,13], a report by Gore and colleagues [14] in 1987 caused many using the PAC to pause and reflect on this approach. Gore and colleagues retrospectively found that the use of this catheter for myocardial infarction complicated by hypotension, shock, or heart failure more than doubled from 1975 to 1984 in the hospitals of their region. In reasonably matched groups, the use of the PAC was associated with higher in-hospital mortality and a longer hospital stay, and there was no difference in the long-term (5-year) survival between the PAC and non-PAC managed groups. Basically, the PAC added little benefit while being associated with a greater length of stay, cost, and death in the management of complicated myocardial infarction in 16 hospitals in mid-eastern Massachusetts. These findings were largely confirmed in a similar patient population (acute coronary syndromes) with a retrospective look at PAC use in the GUSTO II b and III trials [15].

About a decade after the Gore report [14], a retrospective study in critically ill patients admitted with one or more of nine disease categories (cardiac and non-cardiac) to intensive care units in five major medical centers found that PAC placement and use were associated with increased mortality, length of stay, and cost [16].

The results of prospective, randomized, controlled trials (albeit, in non–heart failure populations) examining the use of the PAC were not published until 15 plus years after the Gore report [14]. The French Pulmonary Artery Catheter Study Group found that the PAC itself did not affect outcomes in patients admitted for septic shock or adult respiratory distress syndrome (ARDS) [17]. The same results were observed in over 1000 critically ill patients randomized to PAC or non-PAC management by the PAC-Man Study Group in the United Kingdom [18]. The PAC was associated with a higher complication rate with no observable benefit in patients studied by the ARDS Clinical Trials Network [19]. No benefit was apparent in high-risk surgical patients randomized to PAC or non-PAC management by the Canadian Critical Care Clinical Trials Group [20].

At the turn of the millennium, there were no prospective, randomized, controlled studies investigating the use of the PAC to evaluate and manage heart failure, and, at this point, many of the heart failure specialists in the United States had become polarized into PAC-useful and PAC-useless camps. In 1997, the National Heart, Lung, and Blood Institute and the US Food and Drug Administration conducted a workshop on the study and use of the PAC in this clinical condition. A consensus report from this workshop was published [21] and eventually led to the performance of the Evaluation Study of Congestive Heart Failure and Pulmonary Artery Catheterization and Effectiveness (ESCAPE) trial.

ESCAPE trial

The ESCAPE trial performed in 2000 to 2003 and published in 2005 [22] was a landmark study. It evaluated the use of the PAC in patients hospitalized for advanced heart failure, namely, patients for whom the PAC could be indicated and for whom the PAC would potentially be beneficial. A total of 433 patients hospitalized at 26 study centers for heart failure were randomized into those managed with clinical assessment alone (n = 218) and those managed with clinical assessment plus data attained from PAC placement (n = 215). A comparison of baseline clinical and laboratory variables indicated that the two management groups were well matched. The advanced stage of heart failure in this study population was supported by the following values (PAC and non-PAC groups, respectively): mean left ventricular ejection fractions of 19 ± 7 and 20 ± 6%, blood urea nitrogen (BUN) values of 34 ± 21 and 36 ± 24 mg/dL, serum creatinine of 1.5 ± 0.6 mg/dL in each group, brain natriuretic peptide (BNP) of 974 ± 1216 and 1018 ± 1400 pg/mmol, and, for those who could ambulate, a peak VO_2 of 10.2 ± 3.9 and 9.9 ± 2.9 mL/kg/min and a 6-minute walk 390 ± 400 and 437 ± 431 feet. For the PAC group, the baseline mean right atrial pressure was 14 ± 10 mm Hg, pulmonary artery occlusive pressure 25 ± 9 mm Hg, and cardiac index 1.9 ± 0.6 L/min/m².

The ESCAPE investigators found no difference between the two management groups in the primary endpoint, namely, days alive out of the hospital (Fig. 1). Subgroup analyses also did not uncover differences, although centers with the highest enrollment showed a trend toward improved outcomes in the PAC group, but the difference was not statistically significant. A host of secondary endpoints did not differ between the two groups, with a trend in favor of PAC management for functional assessment (6-minute walk) during the index hospitalization and as shown on Minnesota Living with Heart Failure testing 1 month following discharge. More patients in the PAC group experienced adverse events (21.9% versus 11.5%, P = .04), some of which were attributable to the PAC (eg, infection).

In short, the results of the ESCAPE trial support the view that the PAC should no longer be considered a standard or routine approach in the management of patients hospitalized for advanced or decompensated chronic heart failure; however, the major caveats of this trial must be entered into any conclusions drawn from it. First, patients who the investigators thought must receive a PAC for optimal management were excluded from randomization and study. Second,

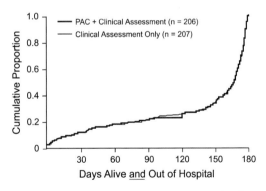

Fig. 1. The primary outcome measure, namely, days well (alive and not in hospital), of the patients in the ESCAPE trial is shown. Early deaths are represented along the left side of the curves and patients surviving to 6 months toward the right. The primary outcome curves of the two treatment groups are nearly identical and statistically the same. Abbreviations: PAC = Swan-Ganz pulmonary artery catheter. (*Adapted from* ESCAPE Investigators and ESCAPE Study Coordinators. Evaluation study of congestive heart failure and pulmonary artery effectiveness: the ESCAPE trial. JAMA 2005; 294:1629; with permission.)

the study involved seasoned physician investigators who were highly experienced in evaluating and managing heart failure patients; therefore, these investigators were able to bring these talents to bear on the management of the clinical assessment alone study group without the dire need for PAC data to guide them. On the other hand, perhaps the PAC, its insertion, and the interpretation of its data also benefited from the same investigators, although the trial, unfortunately, did not record whether the various insertion operators were experienced with the technique or their level of training. Lastly, no standard (or even proven effective) therapies were linked to PAC use or specifically directed by protocol for PAC data in this study group. Each investigator was free to select therapies that were believed to be an optimal intervention for the patient at that point in time. The PAC itself did not manage the patient; the doctors did, resulting in similar interventions for both treatment groups.

Where did we go wrong and what have we learned?

Although the Swan-Ganz PAC is no longer regarded as a routine device to guide the management of heart failure, complicated myocardial infarction, or other critical illnesses, one should not forget the lessons learned from the PAC era. Use of the PAC over many years has led to a better overall understanding and categorization of central hemodynamics in heart failure, myocardial infarction, circulatory shock of all types, complicated pulmonary diseases, and various forms of pulmonary edema. Furthermore, more effective therapies and the rationale for these therapies in managing various critical conditions evolved out of the PAC era. The PAC led to a more comprehensive risk stratification and management of complicated acute myocardial infarction. The PAC provided information regarding the hemodynamic course over time for various threatening cardiovascular conditions (eg, heart failure, pulmonary hypertension). The PAC brought the laboratory concepts of ventricular preload and afterload to the bedside and provided the underpinning for ventricular unloading as a therapeutic means of favorably influencing short- and long-term cardiac function, myocardial remodeling, and the clinical course of heart failure. The PAC provided precise hemodynamic characterization of a wide spectrum of agents developed to enhance cardiac performance and cardiac output and to reduce ventricular diastolic pressures, wall stress, and valvular

insufficiency. The PAC taught us the limitations of acute hemodynamic responses to pharmacologic agents in predicting their long-term responses and clinical outcomes during chronic administration. The PAC better defined the central hemodynamic responses to exercise in health and disease and the effects of interventions on these responses. Perhaps the most noteworthy and lasting consequence of the PAC era was the enhancement of the bedside evaluation and diagnostic skills of two generations of heart failure specialists who were frequently in the position during that era to directly and simultaneously associate a patient's hemodynamic findings with the clinical and physical aspects of their presentation. The PAC was instrumental in spawning the discipline and specialty of heart failure.

The PAC itself does not manage or treat patients; these tasks are still in the decision and performance domains of the physician and the therapeutic tools he or she selects. For many critical illnesses, the limitation is not the PAC but the shortcomings of therapies for the illness and of the interventions used to treat the hemodynamic derangements defined by the PAC. A tenuous link in PAC use remains the involved physician, namely, the person who serves as the operator placing the catheter, the interpreter of the PAC data, and the effector converting the data to proper intervention. Basically, the PAC is only as good as the physician using it and the interventions he or she directs at the information it renders.

Some of the decline in clinical use of the PAC is related to the fact that much of the information needed to effectively treat heart failure and related conditions can be gleaned or reasonably estimated from careful bedside examination and proper interpretation and understanding of pathobiologic and laboratory markers (eg, BNP, serum BUN, creatinine, bicarbonate, and chloride), echocardiography, and other technical developments (eg, impedance cardiography) [23,24]. On the other hand, these modalities are not typically available for use on a continuous basis (or at 2:00 AM) for several successive days.

Complications of the pulmonary artery catheter: the dark side

The Swan-Ganz PAC is considerably more complicated than the commonly employed central venous catheter, and almost every complication one can imagine for the PAC has been reported. Although not absolutely proven by systematic study, safe and proficient placement of the catheter and proper interpretation of the waveforms remain the biggest challenge and are closely related to the skill and experience of the operator interpreter [25]. Misidentification and misinterpretation of waveforms often lead to inappropriate therapies.

It is always disconcerting to witness a scene in which a patient resides under sterile drapes for 45 minutes or longer as the venous access needle or the PAC is passed from intern to resident to cardiology fellow following several unsuccessful attempts at insertion and placement by each. Although learning basic invasive techniques is a major objective of house staff-training programs, the PAC is a cardiac catheter, and its insertion should be performed under the guidance of one well experienced with the procedure. An experienced operator should ideally perform the procedure on the most ill patients for optimal proficiency, safety, and use.

Adverse events associated with placement of the PAC range from local pain, infection, or hemorrhage at the insertion site to death [14–20,22,25–38]. Other reported adverse events include systemic arterial puncture and entry, pneumothorax, conduction block, atrial and ventricular dysrhythmias, thrombus formation with venous occlusion, embolization, pulmonary injury and infarction, aseptic and infectious endocarditis, septicemia and septic shock, knotting and entanglement of the catheter, displacement of pacing electrodes, right-sided heart or pulmonary artery perforation or rupture, superior vena cava syndrome, and, amazingly, intrathecal insertion. These complications can be expected to occur more frequently in non-ideal settings, during urgent placement, with inexperienced operators and bedside care givers, and related situations.

Guidelines and recommendations

In concert with the already evolving clinical impression regarding the PAC, the principal (and principle) conclusion of the ESCAPE trial [22] was as follows: "Based on ESCAPE, there is no indication for the routine use of PACs to adjust therapy during hospitalization for decompensation of chronic heart failure."

The 2005 American Heart Association/American College of Cardiology (AHA/ACC) updated guidelines for chronic heart failure [39], published 15 days before the results of the ESCAPE trial appeared in print, had already relegated PAC use to a class IIB indication in patients with refractory end-stage heart failure (stage D heart, New York Heart Association functional class IV). The guidelines specifically state the following: "Class IIB 1. Pulmonary artery catheter placement may be reasonable to guide therapy in patients with refractory end-stage HF and persistently severe symptoms (Level of Evidence: C)." Several members of the AHA/ACC update committee were also investigators in the ESCAPE Trial.

Where does the Swan-Ganz pulmonary artery catheter stand in 2007?

Considerations for the current use of the PAC are listed in Box 1. Centers and operators

---

Box 1. Considerations for use of the Swan-Ganz PAC in heart failure and related conditions in the post-ESCAPE era

1. Evaluation of pulmonary artery pressure, pulmonic vascular resistance, and pharmacologic responsiveness of pulmonary vasculature in patients undergoing evaluation for cardiac transplantation and, occasionally, for placement of an LVAD.
2. Clarification of pulmonary versus cardiac origin of pulmonary hypertension.
3. Evaluation of therapies (agents and dosing) for primary pulmonary hypertension.
4. Assessment of cardiac versus non-cardiac causes of pulmonary edema.
5. Application of interventions needed to treat the patient with persistent hypotension-hypoperfusion following adequate (or more) fluid resuscitation and initial therapeutic efforts.
6. Determination of whether dyspnea may have a cardiac source in the patient with chronic lung disease.
7. Evaluation in select patients of problematic symptom-limited exercise performance or activity intolerance.
8. Hemodynamic characterization in the research and development of therapeutic agents for critical and acute cardiac care.

experienced with its use are the preferred conditions for PAC use. The PAC should be considered when a patient's imminently threatening cardiovascular condition does not respond adequately to standard interventions. Examples include persistent systemic hypotension and hypoperfusion following adequate (or more) fluid resuscitation and initial pharmacotherapeutic attempts, or when apparently contradictory clinical and laboratory findings confuse or delay an effective therapeutic plan in this setting. The PAC remains clinically useful in separating cardiac from pulmonary origins of pulmonary hypertension and in the pharmacotherapeutics of primary pulmonary hypertension. This device can be helpful in distinguishing cardiogenic from non-cardiogenic pulmonary edema and in determining whether dyspnea has a cardiac explanation in patients with chronic lung disease and inconclusive BNP levels. The PAC remains the principal means of assessing pulmonary vascular resistance and reactivity in patients undergoing evaluation for cardiac transplantation and, occasionally, for placement of a left ventricular assist device (LVAD). The PAC with its ability to provide continuous, precise hemodynamic information will remain a reliable device in the research and development of therapeutic agents for critical and acute cardiac care.

Summary

A special catheter was developed 35 to 40 years ago for intensive and cardiac care units to allow bedside placement and continuous monitoring and recording of right-sided heart, pulmonary artery, and wedge pressures and reasonably accurate determinations of cardiac output. This balloon-tip, flow-directed, multilumen, thermodilution PAC is generally known as the Swan-Ganz catheter. It enjoyed widespread use as a research and clinical device for about two to three decades, particularly in the study and management of myocardial infarction, heart failure, pulmonary edema, shock states, cardiac surgery, and other critical conditions. Over the past 15 years, several controlled trials have shown that the Swan-Ganz catheter has limited value in achieving better outcomes for most of these conditions. For heart failure, the ESCAPE trial arrived at a similar result and conclusion. This trial and current guidelines now advocate that the Swan-Ganz catheter should no longer be regarded as a routine approach in the management of advanced heart failure.

In its wake, the Swan-Ganz PAC has left a legacy of better understanding of the hemodynamics of heart failure and related illnesses and of the management and therapeutics to address these conditions. Considerations for the clinical application of this catheter in the post-ESCAPE era are presented herein.

References

[1] Forssmann W. The catheterization of the right side of the heart. Klin Wochenschr 1929;45:2085–7.

[2] Cournand A, Ranges HA. Catheterization of the right auricle in man. Proc Soc Exp Biol Med 1941; 46:462–6.

[3] Cournand A, Lauson HD, Bloomfield RA, et al. Recording of right heart pressures in man. Proc Soc Exp Biol Med 1944;55:34–6.

[4] Hellems HK, Haynes FW, Dexter L. Pulmonary 'capillary' pressure in man. J Appl Physiol 1949;2: 24–9.

[5] Connolly DC, Kirklin JW, Wood EH. The relationship between pulmonary artery wedge pressure and left atrial pressure in man. Circ Res 1954;2:434–40.

[6] Swan HJC, Ganz W, Forrester J, et al. Catheterization of the heart in man with use of a flow-directed balloon-tipped catheter. N Engl J Med 1979;283: 447–51.

[7] Ganz W, Donoso R, Marcus HS, et al. A new technique for measurement of cardiac output by thermodilution in man. Am J Cardiol 1971;27:392–6.

[8] Desch CE, Magorien RD, Triffon DW, et al. The development of pharmacodynamic tolerance to prazosin in congestive heart failure. Am J Cardiol 1979;44: 1178–82.

[9] Packer M, Medina N, Yushak M, et al. Hemodynamic patterns of response during long-term captopril therapy for severe heart failure. Circulation 1983;68:803–12.

[10] Leier CV, Patrick TJ, Hermiller J, et al. Nifedipine in congestive heart failure: effects on resting and exercise hemodynamics and regional blood flow. Am Heart J 1984;108:1461–7.

[11] Massie BM, Kramer BL, Topic N. Lack of relationship between the short-term hemodynamic effects of captopril and subsequent clinical responses. Circulation 1984;69:1135–41.

[12] Berlauk JF, Abrams JH, Gilmour IJ, et al. Preoperative optimization of cardiovascular hemodynamics improves outcome in peripheral vascular surgery: a prospective randomized clinical trial. Ann Surg 1991;214:289–99.

[13] Ivanov R, Allen J, Calvin JE. The incidence of major morbidity in critically ill patients managed with pulmonary artery catheters: a meta-analysis. Crit Care Med 2000;28:615–9.

[14] Gore JM, Goldberg RJ, Spodick DH, et al. A community-wide assessment of the use of pulmonary

artery catheters in patients with acute myocardial infarction. Chest 1987;92:721–7.

[15] Cohen MG, Kelly RV, Kong DF, et al. Pulmonary artery catheterization in acute coronary syndromes: insights from the GUSTO II b and GUSTO III trials. Am J Med 2005;118:482–8.

[16] Connor AF Jr, Speroff T, Dawson NV, et al. SUPPORT Investigators. The effectiveness of right heart catheterization in the initial care of critically ill patients. JAMA 1996;276:889–97.

[17] French Pulmonary Artery Catheter Study Group. Early use of the pulmonary artery catheter and outcomes in patients with shock and acute respiratory distress syndrome: a randomized controlled trial. JAMA 2003;290:2713–20.

[18] PAC-Man Study Collaboration. Assessment of the clinical effectiveness of pulmonary artery catheters in management of patients in intensive care (PAC-Man): a randomized controlled trial. Lancet 2005; 366:472–7.

[19] National Heart, Lung, and Blood Institute Acute Respiratory Distress Syndrome (ARDS) Clinical Trials Network. Pulmonary-artery versus central venous catheter to guide treatment of acute lung injury. N Engl J Med 2006;354:2213–24.

[20] Canadian Critical Care Clinical Trials Group. A randomized, controlled trial of the use of pulmonary catheters in high-risk surgical patients. N Engl J Med 2003;348:5–14.

[21] Bernard GR, Sopko G, Cerra F, et al. Pulmonary artery catheter and clinical outcomes: National Heart, Lung, and Blood Institute and Food and Drug Administration workshop report. Consensus statement. JAMA 2000;283:2568–72.

[22] ESCAPE Investigators and ESCAPE Study Coordinators. Evaluation study of congestive heart failure and pulmonary artery effectiveness: the ESCAPE trial. JAMA 2005;294:1625–33.

[23] Leier CV. Nuggets, pearls, and clinical vignettes of master heart failure clinicians. Part 2. The physical examination. Congest Heart Fail 2001;7: 297–308.

[24] Oh JK. Echocardiography as a noninvasive Swan-Ganz catheter. Circulation 2005;111:3192–4.

[25] Raper R, Sibbald WJ. Misled by the wedge? The Swan-Ganz catheter and left ventricular preload. Chest 1986;89:427–34.

[26] Connors AF, Castele RJ, Farhat NZ, et al. Complications of right heart catheterization: a prospective autopsy study. Chest 1985;88:567–72.

[27] Rowley KM, Clubb KS, Smith GJW, et al. Right-sided infective endocarditis as a consequence of flow-directed pulmonary-artery catheterization. N Engl J Med 1984;311:1152–6.

[28] Iberti TJ, Benjamin E, Gruppi L, et al. Ventricular arrhythmias during pulmonary artery catheterization in the intensive care unit. Am J Med 1985;78:451–4.

[29] Lange HW, Galliani CA, Edwards JE. Local complications associated with indwelling Swan-Ganz catheters: autopsy study of 36 cases. Am J Cardiol 1983; 52:1108–11.

[30] Sprung CL, Pozen RG, Rozanski JJ, et al. Advanced ventricular arrhythmias during bedside pulmonary artery catheterization. Am J Med 1982;72:203–8.

[31] Swan HJ, Ganz W. Complications with flow-directed balloon-tipped catheters. Ann Intern Med 1979;91:494.

[32] Santiago SM, Williams AJ. Acute superior vena cava syndrome after Swan-Ganz catheterization. Chest 1986;89:319–20.

[33] Patil AR. Risk of right bundle-branch block and complete heart block during pulmonary artery catheterization. Crit Care Med 1990;18:122–3.

[34] Mermel LA, McCormick RD, Springman SR, et al. The pathogenesis and epidemiology of catheter-related infection with pulmonary artery Swan-Ganz catheters: a prospective study utilizing molecular subtyping. Am J Med 1991;91:197S–205S.

[35] Kelly TF Jr, Morris GC Jr, Crawford ES, et al. Perforation of the pulmonary artery with Swan-Ganz catheters: diagnosis and surgical management. Ann Surg 1981;193:686–92.

[36] Urschel JD, Myerowitz PD. Catheter-induced pulmonary artery rupture in the setting of cardiopulmonary bypass. Ann Thorac Surg 1993;56:585–9.

[37] Nagai K, Kemmotsu O. An inadvertent insertion of a Swan-Ganz catheter into the intrathecal space. Anesthesiology 1985;62:848–9.

[38] Bossert T, Gummert JF, Bittner HB, et al. Swan-Ganz catheter-induced severe complications in cardiac surgery: right ventricular perforation, knotting, and rupture of a pulmonary artery. J Card Surg 2006;21:292–5.

[39] Hunt SA, Abraham WT, Chin MH, et al. Writing Committee to Update the 2001 Guidelines for the Evaluation and Management of Heart Failure. ACC/AHA 2005 Guideline Update for the Diagnosis and Management of Chronic Heart Failure in the Adult—Summary Article. Circulation 2005;112: 1825–52.

CARDIOLOGY
CLINICS

Cardiol Clin 25 (2007) 573–580

ELSEVIER
SAUNDERS

Anti-angiotensin Therapy: New Perspectives

Kumudha Ramasubbu, MD[a],*, Douglas L. Mann, MD[b],
Anita Deswal, MD, MPH[a]

[a]Micheal E. DeBakey Veterans Affairs Medical Center, Houston, TX, USA
[b]Baylor College of Medicine, Houston, TX, USA

Activation of the renin-angiotensin system (RAS) plays an important role in the pathogenesis of heart failure. Thus, strategies for the treatment of heart failure have focused on agents that block the RAS. Angiotensin-converting-enzyme (ACE) inhibitors are established for the treatment of heart failure. More recently, the role of angiotensin receptor blockers (ARBs) in heart failure therapy has been better defined. This article examines the rationale and role of ARBs in the treatment of patients with heart failure based on evidence from clinical trials.

Rationale for use of angiotensin receptor blockers in heart failure

Activation of the RAS is central to the pathophysiology of heart failure. The deleterious effects of RAS are mediated primarily through the neurohormone angiotensin II [1]. The RAS can be inhibited at various levels of the enzyme cascade as shown in Fig. 1. ACE inhibitors block the ACE, which converts angiotensin I to angiotensin II, thus reducing the angiotensin II that is available to stimulate the AT_1 and AT_2 receptors. However, the use of ACE inhibitors does not lead to complete suppression of angiotensin II levels in patients with heart failure, and levels of angiotensin II gradually increase despite chronic ACE inhibitor therapy [2–5]. Various pathways have been proposed to explain this "escape" from ACE inhibition. First, the competitive inhibition of ACE results in an increase in renin and

angiotensin I, which may overcome the blockade of this enzyme [6]. Second, angiotensin I is converted to angiotensin II through alternative, non-ACE enzymatic pathways using chymase, kallikrein, cathepsin G, and tonin [5,7,8]. The chymase pathway appears to be responsible for the majority of angiotensin II production in human vasculature, with only 30% to 40% of angiotensin II being produced via the ACE pathway [9,10]. Moreover, one study demonstrated that ACE inhibitors block only 13% of human cardiac angiotensin II production, whereas 87% of the angiotensin II is produced by non-ACE pathways [11]. On the premise of such observations, angiotensin receptor antagonists were developed to enable a more complete inhibition of angiotensin II activity by directly blocking the AT_1 receptor.

Of note, ACE inhibitors appear to exert favorable effects partially by increasing bradykinin levels by blocking the breakdown of bradykinin by kininase II, which is identical to ACE (see Fig. 1). Potential beneficial effects of bradykinin in heart failure include vasodilation through the release of nitric oxide and prostaglandin, and antimitotic and antithrombotic actions [12]. However, bradykinin is also likely responsible for the adverse reaction of cough with the use of ACE inhibitors [13], and it stimulates the release of catecholamines, which can be arrhythmogenic [14]. Compared with ACE inhibitors, ARBs do not appear to potentiate bradykinin actions. These differences in neurohormonal modulation and adverse effects indicate that the benefits and risks of ACE inhibitors and ARBs may differ. Furthermore, these observations suggest that the actions of ACE inhibitors and ARBs may be complementary and thus provide a rationale to evaluate

* Corresponding author.
E-mail address: kumudhar@bcm.edu (K. Ramasubbu).

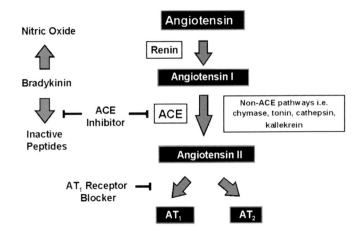

Fig. 1. Activation of the renin angiotensin system. Angiotensinogen is converted to angiotensin I by renin. Angiotensin I can be converted to angiotensin II by the angiotensin converting enzyme (ACE) and non–ACE-dependent pathways. Angiotensin II exerts its biological effects by binding to type I (AT$_1$) and type II (AT$_2$) angiotensin receptors. (*Modified from* Mann DL, Deswal A, Bozkurt B, et al. New therapeutics for chronic heart failure. Annu Rev Med 2002;53:59–74; with permission. Reprinted with permission from the Annual Review of Medicine, Volume 53 © 2002 by Annual Reviews www.annualreviews.org <file://www.annualreviews.org>.)

a combination of the two classes of agents in patients with heart failure. Therefore, the addition of an ARB to ACE inhibitor may offer more complete AT$_1$ blockade than could be achieved with ACE inhibition alone, while preserving the beneficial effects of bradykinin potentiation offered by ACE inhibitors.

On the basis of these theoretical considerations, as well as promising results from experimental and clinical data, large-scale clinical trials were developed to assess the beneficial effect of ARBs as alternatives to ACE inhibitors and the beneficial effect of the ACE inhibitor/ARB combination compared with ACE inhibitors alone in patients with heart failure. The clinical trial evidence available to date on the use of ARBs in patients with chronic heart failure is reviewed here.

Angiotensin receptor blockers in chronic heart failure

Angiotensin receptor blockers as alternatives to angiotensin-converting-enzyme inhibitors in patients with chronic heart failure

Several trials compared the efficacy of ARBs to ACE inhibitors in chronic heart failure. The Evaluation of Losartan In The Evaluation of Losartan In The Elderly I (ELITE I) trial compared the effects of losartan and captopril on renal function and tolerability in elderly patients with

symptomatic heart failure secondary to left ventricular systolic dysfunction [15]. The patients were randomized to either captopril or losartan for 48 weeks (Table 1). There was no significant difference in the frequency of the primary endpoint of a persistent increase of greater than or equal to 0.3 mg/dL in serum creatinine, between the losartan and captopril groups (10.5% in each group). However, a trend toward lower mortality or hospital admission for heart failure was noted in the losartan group (9.4% versus 13.2%, $P = .075$), with the benefit primarily driven by a 46% decrease in all-cause mortality based on a small number of events that were not part of the primary study endpoint. As a result, a second, larger trial of 3152 patients—the Evaluation of Losartan In The Elderly II (ELITE II)—was initiated to compare the effects of captopril and losartan on mortality in heart failure patients similar to those enrolled in ELITE I [16]. However, ELITE II showed no significant difference in all-cause mortality (17.7% versus 15.9% for losartan and captopril, respectively; hazard ratio [HR] 1.13, 95% CI, 0.95–1.35, $P = .16$) or sudden death or resuscitated arrests (9.0 versus 7.3%, $P = .08$) between the two treatment groups [16]. Thus, treatment with ARB was not superior to ACE inhibition; in fact, a trend toward improved outcomes was noted with ACE inhibitors. This finding may suggest that the bradykinin effects of ACE inhibitors played a role in this marginal benefit with ACE inhibitors over ARBs. However, it

Table 1
Clinical trials of angiotensin receptor blockers in chronic heart failure

Trial; number of patients (n)	Study population	Study drug	Comparator
ELITE I [15] n = 722	LVEF≤40% NYHA II-III≥65 years	Losartan 50 mg daily	Captopril 50 three times daily
ELITE II [16] n = 3152	LVEF≤40% NYHA II-III≥60 years	Losartan 50 mg daily	Captopril 50 three times daily
CHARM-Alternative [18] n = 2028	LVEF≤40% NYHA II-IV intolerance to ACE inhibitors	Candesartan 32 mg daily	Placebo
Val-HeFT [21] n = 5010	LVEF<40% NYHA II-IV 93% on ACE inhibitors	Valsartan 160 mg twice daily	Placebo
CHARM-Added [22] n = 2458	LVEF≤40% NYHA II-IV all patients on ACE inhibitors	Candesartan 32 mg daily	Placebo

Abbreviations: ACE, angiotensin-converting-enzyme; CHARM, Candesartan in Heart failure: Assessment of Reduction in Mortality and Morbidity; ELITE, Evaluation of Losartan In The Elderly; LVEF, left ventricular ejection fraction; NYHA, New York Heart Association; Val-HeFT, Valsartan in Heart failure Trial.

has been suggested that the dose of losartan used in the ELITE trials (50 mg daily) may not fully block AT_1 receptors throughout the 24-hour dosing interval and that higher doses may have been more effective [17].

In a further large-scale trial, the Candesartan in Heart Failure: Assessment of Reduction in Mortality and Morbidity (CHARM)-Alternative trial, patients with symptomatic systolic heart failure and history of intolerance to ACE inhibitors were randomized to either candesartan or to placebo (see Table 1) [18]. Patients treated with candesartan demonstrated a significant 23% reduction in the primary composite outcome of cardiovascular mortality or heart failure hospitalization (HR 0.77, 95% CI, 0.67–0.89; $P = .0004$) as well as a significant reduction in the individual endpoints of cardiovascular death, heart failure hospitalization, and other cardiovascular morbidity. Interestingly, the 23% reduction in cardiovascular mortality and heart failure hospitalizations is similar to the 26% reduction in these outcomes reported in clinical trials evaluating the use of ACE inhibitors in patients with left ventricular systolic dysfunction [19,20].

Further support for ARBs as an alternative in patients with heart failure intolerant to ACE inhibitors was provided by results of the Valsartan in Heart Failure Trial (Val-HeFT) in a small subgroup of patients who were not on ACE inhibitors at baseline (see below) [21]. On the basis of the results of ELITE II trial, the CHARM-Alternative study, and the subgroup analysis in the Val-

HeFT trial, ACE inhibitors continue to be the recommended agents of choice for patients with heart failure and depressed left ventricular systolic function. That said, ARBs—specifically candesartan and valsartan—confer significant benefit on mortality and morbidity in patients with heart failure who are intolerant of ACE inhibitors and therefore offer a good alternative strategy in these patients.

Angiotensin receptor blockers in addition to angiotensin-converting-enzyme inhibitors in patients with chronic heart failure

Theoretically, the more complete angiotensin II inhibition using a combination of ACE inhibitors and ARBs in patients with heart failure may translate into improved clinical outcomes. This concept led to the development of clinical trials evaluating the efficacy of ARBs as add-on therapy to ACE inhibitors in patients with left ventricular systolic dysfunction and symptomatic heart failure. Two large clinical trials in patients with heart failure, the Val-HeFT and the CHARM-Added trial, evaluated the impact of adding ARBs to ACE inhibitors on morbidity and mortality. In Val-HeFT, patients with left ventricular systolic dysfunction and New York Heart Association (NYHA) class II-IV heart failure were randomized to receive valsartan (goal dose of 160 mg twice daily) or placebo (see Table 1). At baseline, patients were already receiving standard therapy for heart failure, which included ACE inhibitors in 93% and beta blockers in 35% of patients [21]. At follow-up, the first primary endpoint, mortality, was similar in the two groups. The second primary endpoint, combination of mortality and morbidity, was 13.2% lower in patients treated with valsartan ($P = .009$). The benefit was primarily attributed to a 24% reduction in the rate of hospitalizations for heart failure in patients taking valsartan. Improvements were also seen with valsartan in several secondary endpoints, including left ventricular ejection fraction, signs and symptoms of heart failure, and quality of life.

Subgroup analysis revealed that a small subgroup of 366 patients (7%) who were not receiving ACE inhibitors received maximal benefit with valsartan: a 33% reduction in mortality and a 49% decrease in mortality and morbidity compared with placebo. This is in contrast to the lack of morbidity and mortality benefit with valsartan observed in the overall trial in patients already receiving background ACE inhibitor therapy (HR, 0.92; $P = .0965$). However, a modest favorable trend was noted in the group receiving an ACE inhibitor, largely driven by the patients receiving less than the recommended dose of an ACE inhibitor [21]. In summary, when added to standard therapy, valsartan has no overall effect on mortality and produced a modest reduction in morbidity. However, this benefit was much larger in patients not receiving concomitant ACE inhibitor therapy, but was not statistically significant in those who were already taking ACE inhibitors.

In a second trial, the CHARM-Added Trial, 2458 patients with symptomatic systolic heart failure already on an ACE inhibitor were randomized to either candesartan or placebo (see Table 1) [22]. Baseline therapy included beta blockers in 55%, spironolactone in 17%, and diuretics in 90% of patients. After a median follow-up of 41 months, 38% of patients in the candesartan group and 42% of patients in the placebo group experienced the primary outcome of cardiovascular death or heart failure hospitalization (unadjusted HR 0.85; 95% CI, 0.75–0.96; $P = .01$) as a result of a significant reduction in cardiovascular mortality as well as heart failure hospitalizations in the candesartan group. Candesartan also had a significant beneficial effect on several secondary cardiovascular outcomes.

Taken together, the results of Val-HeFT and CHARM-Added suggest that there is a reduction in heart failure hospitalizations when an ARB is added to an ACE inhibitor. However, the impact of adding an ARB to an ACE inhibitor on mortality is less clear. That is, although there was a significant benefit on cardiovascular mortality in the CHARM-Added trial, there was only a trend toward benefit for all-cause mortality. Moreover, there was no mortality benefit in the Val-HeFT study. The reasons for the discrepancy between these two studies is not clear, but may include differences in the pharmakokinetics of valsartan and candesartan, differences in the effective dosages that were used, and differences in baseline patient characteristics. Interestingly, patients in CHARM-Added had more severe heart failure (about 73% with NYHA class III) than in Val HeFT (about 62% with NYHA class II). On the basis of the aggregate results of these trials, the current American College of Cardiology/American Heart Association guidelines recommend the addition of ARBs to ACE inhibitors in patients who continue to have symptoms of heart failure despite receiving target doses of ACE inhibitors and beta blockers, or in patients with heart failure who are on ACE inhibitors but are unable to tolerate beta blockers [23].

Of note, a higher rate of discontinuation of the study drug was reported for worsening renal function or hyperkalemia in patients on ARB compared with those on placebo in the Val-HeFT and CHARM trials [21,22]. In the CHARM study, discontinuation for increase in serum creatinine was 7.8% in the candesartan arm compared with 4.1% in the placebo group ($P = .0001$). Similarly, drug discontinuation for hyperkalemia was significantly higher in the candesartan arm (3.4%) compared with the placebo arm (0.7%, $P < .0001$). Thus, careful monitoring of renal function and serum potassium while initiating and up-titrating doses of ARBs is recommended.

Potential explanations for discrepant clinical trial results of angiotensin receptor blockers in heart failure

Thus far, clinical trials evaluating ARBs in patients with heart failure have demonstrated differences in clinical outcomes. Again, the reasons for this discrepancy remain unclear, but may relate to differences in pharmakokinetics and dosage of the ARBs. Although all ARBs block the AT_1 receptor, they differ in pharmacokinetics, including differences in binding characteristics. AT_1 receptor antagonism has been classified as surmountable and insurmountable [6]. With surmountable antagonism, the blockade by the antagonist (ARB) can be overcome with increasing concentrations of the agonist (angiotensin II), whereas with insurmountable antagonism, the blockade by the ARB cannot be overcome with increasing concentrations of angiotensin II. Thus, insurmountable antagonism is associated with a reduction in maximal angiotensin II activity, whereas surmountable antagonism is not. With ARB therapy, plasma angiotensin II concentrations increase as a result of interrupting the negative feedback. Theoretically, more clinical benefit may be expected with the use of an insurmountable AT_1 receptor blocker antagonist, which would not likely to be overcome by higher levels of circulating angiotensin II. Valsartan, irbesartan, candesartan, and an active metabolite of losartan (EXP3174) are insurmountable AT_1 receptor antagonists, whereas losartan is a surmountable antagonist [6]. Moreover, differences exist in the potency of ARBs with respect to their antihypertensive effect. Candesartan has been demonstrated to be the most potent, followed by irbesartan, valsartan, and lastly losartan [1]. Whether these differences in pharmakokinetics contribute to the improved outcomes observed in clinical trials using valsartan or candesartan in heart failure patients compared with those using losartan is, however, not clear.

Another important factor that may play a role in the observed differences in benefits noted between various ARBs is the issue of appropriate dosing and thus degree of RAS inhibition. Choosing the appropriate dose of a therapeutic agent is perhaps as important as choosing the correct therapeutic agent. In trials evaluating the efficacy of an ARB in comparison with an ACE inhibitor, the achievement of comparable RAS inhibition is important. For example, the dosing strategy of 50 mg/d of losartan versus 150 mg/d of captopril favored the use of captopril over losartan in patients with moderate to severe heart failure in the ELITE II trial [16] and also favored captopril in the postmyocardial infarction Optimal Therapy in Myocardial Infarction with the Angiotensin II Antagonist Losartan (OPTIMAAL) trial [24]. In contrast, in trials of patients with hypertensive left ventricular hypertrophy and with diabetic nephropathy, higher doses of losartan up to 100 mg/d were associated with a significant reduction in the incidence of heart failure [25,26], posing the question whether higher doses of losartan may have been more effective in reducing cardiovascular outcomes in OPTIMAAL and ELITE II. In support of this concept, in a second postmyocardial

infarction trial, the VALsartan In Acute myocardial iNfarcTion (VALIANT) trial, a higher dose of valsartan (160 mg twice daily) was used—a dose that is higher than its usual indicated dose in hypertension (160 mg daily)—and demonstrated equivalent benefit compared with captopril. That there were greater reductions in blood pressure and more frequent hypotension-related adverse effects with valsartan in VALIANT compared with losartan in OPTIMAAL also supports more complete RAS blockade at the higher dose of valsartan used in the VALIANT trial.

Similarly, in trials evaluating the addition of an ARB to an ACE inhibitor, it is important to recognize the extent of RAS inhibition with the combination when comparing the results of the trials. For example, VALIANT is the only trial among the ARB trials in which the dose of the ACE inhibitor was titrated up to a maximum target, resulting in a higher dose of ACE inhibitors in VALIANT (mean captopril dose of 117 mg) than in CHARM (mean captopril dose of about 80 mg). This may have decreased the chances to observe the beneficial effect of addition of an ARB in VALIANT. Also, in the combination arm of the VALIANT trial, a lower dose of ARB (80 mg twice daily) was used compared with a higher dose used in the monotherapy arm (160 mg twice daily). The outcomes in the monotherapy arm were comparable to the captopril arm, but no additional benefit was obtained by adding valsartan to captopril in the combination arm. Possibly, the dose of valsartan was not high enough to show a benefit when added to full-dose ACE inhibition. This was in contrast to the CHARM and Val-HeFT trials, which demonstrated improvement in morbidity when higher ARB doses were added to ACE inhibitors [27,28]. Interestingly, in Val-HeFT, a small subgroup of patients who were not receiving ACE inhibitors received maximal benefit with valsartan followed by a modest benefit in those on ACE inhibitors but not beta blockers, and those on beta blockers but not ACE inhibitors. Thus, these observations suggest that a ceiling effect may be reached when employing various neurohormonal therapies. The extent of benefit when adding an ARB appears not only to depend on the ARB dosage, but also on the baseline treatment with other neurohormonal antagonists (beta blockers and ACE inhibitors).

A concerning finding in Val-HeFT was the 42% increase in mortality with valsartan in patients receiving both ACE inhibitor and beta blocker ($P = .009$). A potential explanation proposed for this observation was an excessive inhibition of the neurohormonal system. However, this finding was not substantiated by subsequent trials with ARBs and was thus thought to be a chance finding of multiple subgroup analyses. In the CHARM-Added trial, subgroup analysis revealed benefit of candesartan on the primary outcome in all patients, irrespective of baseline treatment with beta blockers, as well as in patients receiving recommended doses of ACE inhibitors. Regardless, a balance appears to be important between sufficient RAS inhibition to reap clinical outcome benefits on the one side versus not too excessive RAS inhibition that results in more adverse events on the other side. This balance likely needs to be determined on an individual basis based on the patient's blood pressure, renal function, and stage of heart failure. With the current data from the CHARM and Val-HeFT, valsartan and candesartan, at doses used in the clinical trials, are the recommended ARBs for patients with chronic heart failure (Table 2).

Future perspectives/unanswered questions

Several questions remain with respect to RAS inhibition in heart failure. Although the combination of ACE inhibitor and ARB has been demonstrated to result in improved morbidity and mortality, it is unclear whether this is because these two drug classes complement each other's actions, leading to an additive effect, or whether this merely reflects a more complete inhibition of the RAS. If the latter is the case, perhaps higher doses of ARBs may have the same outcome as the combination ACE inhibitors and ARBs. In the treatment of hypertension, the hypothesis of enhanced organ protection with doses higher than those approved by the US Food and Drug Administration is currently being explored in three different studies using 640-mg valsartan, 128-mg candesartan, and 900-mg irbesartan [29].

In patients with moderate to severe heart failure, there are no data to guide the decision of whether to first add an aldosterone receptor blocker (based on the beneficial effect seen in the Randomized Aldactone Evaluation Studies [30]) or an ARB. Given that the combined blockade with ACE inhibitors and ARBs has not demonstrated an incremental effect on the decrease in plasma aldosterone (possibly due to the non-angiotensin aldosterone activating pathways), one might argue that the addition of an aldosterone receptor blocker may be more beneficial than the addition of an ARB to ACE inhibitor therapy [31]. However, it bears emphasis that the safety and efficacy of triple RAS-inhibiting therapy using an ACE inhibitor, an ARB, and an aldosterone antagonist is not known, and is currently not recommended by the American College of Cardiology/American Heart Association guidelines [32].

More recently, the direct renin inhibitor, aliskiren, has been investigated for the treatment of hypertension [33–35]. Since aliskiren inhibits renin, which catalyzes the first step of the RAS cascade, more down-stream products of the RAS will be affected than is the case with ARBs and ACE inhibitors, resulting in a more wide-ranging inhibition of the RAS. Furthermore, the fact that renin has high specificity to one substrate—angiotensinogen—and does not affect bradykinin metabolism may be indicative of fewer side effects and better tolerability. So far, clinical trials evaluating aliskiren in patients with hypertension have demonstrated modest blood pressure reductions with good tolerability with doses up to 300 mg. The role for renin inhibitors in heart failure patients is unclear at this time. Although a more comprehensive blockade of the RAS may be beneficial in heart failure, it is unknown if this may potentially worsen outcomes due to complete inhibition of a compensatory system. Furthermore, in patients with hypertension, although aliskiren suppressed plasma renin activity [33], renin concentration was increased due to loss of feedback inhibition by angiotensin II on renin release. The extent of increase in renin concentration in patients with heart failure, and whether this is associated with further consequences (eg, the overcoming of renin inhibition), remains to be determined. Lastly, the role of renin inhibitors among the other RAS antagonists in heart failure will need to be clarified. The main questions center on incremental clinical benefit and safety of multiple RAS inhibitors, especially with respect to hypotension, hyperkalemia, and renal insufficiency. The

Table 2
Angiotensin receptor blockers evaluated in heart failure trials

Drug	Recommended starting dosage	Recommended target dosage
Valsartan[a]	40 mg twice daily	160 mg twice daily
Candesartan[a]	4 mg daily	32 mg daily
Losartan	25 mg daily	50 mg daily

[a] Recommended angiotensin receptor blockers in patients with heart failure.

Aliskiren Observation of Heart Failure Treatment trial is in the planning stages and will hopefully shed some light on these questions.

Summary

On the basis of the results of clinical trial, there is a role for ARBs in the treatment of patients with chronic heart failure. However, as a result of the much larger clinical experience as well as the lower cost of ACE inhibitors compared with ARBs, ACE inhibitors continue to be the preferred agents for RAS inhibition in heart failure patients. In patients intolerant of ACE inhibitors, the ARBs valsartan and candesartan (at doses used in clinical trials) are recommended as alternative agents (see Table 2). The addition of ARBs to ACE inhibitor therapy may be considered in patients who continue to have heart failure symptoms or uncontrolled hypertension, despite recommended doses of ACE inhibitors and beta blockers. Several questions with respect to RAS antagonism in heart failure remain to be addressed. To date, in patients with moderate to severe heart failure despite therapy with an ACE inhibitor and a beta blocker, it is unclear whether an aldosterone inhibitor or an ARB should be added first. Also, the efficacy and safety of combining ACE inhibitors, ARBs, and aldosterone receptor antagonists, in addition to beta blockers and the role of the renin inhibitor aliskiren in heart failure, remain to be determined.

References

[1] Burnier M, Brunner HR. Angiotensin II receptor antagonists. Lancet 2000;355:637–45.

[2] Jorde UP, Ennezat PV, Lisker J, et al. Maximally recommended doses of angiotensin-converting enzyme (ACE) inhibitors do not completely prevent ACE-mediated formation of angiotensin II in chronic heart failure. Circulation 2000;101:844–6.

[3] Kawamura M, Imanashi M, Matsushima Y, et al. Circulating angiotensin II levels under repeated administration of lisinopril in normal subjects. Clin Exp Pharmacol Physiol 1992;19:547–53.

[4] de Gasparo M, Levens N. Does blockade of angiotensin II receptors offer clinical benefits over inhibition of angiotensin-converting enzyme? Pharmacol Toxicol 1998;82:257–71.

[5] Wolny A, Clozel J-P, Rein J, et al. Functional and biochemical analysis of angiotensin II-forming pathways in the human heart. Circ Res 1997;80:219–27.

[6] McConnaughey MM, McConnaughey JS, Ingenito AJ. Practical considerations of the pharmacology of angiotensin receptor blockers. J Clin Pharmacol 1999;39:547–59.

[7] Petrie MC, Padmanabhan N, McDonald JE, et al. Angiotensin converting enzyme (ACE) and non-ACE dependent angiotensin II generation in resistance arteries from patients with heart failure and coronary heart disease. J Am Coll Cardiol 2001;37:1056–61.

[8] Dzau VJ. Multiple pathways of angiotensin production in the blood vessel wall: evidence, possibilities and hypotheses. J Hypertens 1989;7:933–6.

[9] Okunishi H, Oka Y, Shiota N, et al. Marked species-difference in the vascular angiotensin II-forming pathways: humans versus rodents. Jpn J Pharmacol 1993;62:207–10.

[10] Liao Y, Husain A. The chymase-angiotensin system in humans: biochemistry, molecular biology and potential role in cardiovascular diseases. Can J Cardiol 1995;11(Suppl F):13F–9F.

[11] Urata H, Healy B, Stewart RW, et al. Angiotensin II-forming pathways in normal and failing human hearts. Circ Res 1990;66:883–90.

[12] Gavras I. Bradykinin-mediated effects of ACE inhibition. Kidney Int 1992;42:1020–9.

[13] Israili ZH, Hall WD. Cough and angioneurotic edema associated with angiotensin-converting enzyme inhibitor therapy. A review of the literature and pathophysiology. Ann Intern Med 1992;117:234–42.

[14] Rump LC, Oberhauser V, Schwertfeger E, et al. Experimental evidence to support ELITE. Lancet 1998;351:644–5.

[15] Pitt B, Segal R, Martinez FA, et al. Randomized trial of losartan versus captopril in patients over 65 with heart failure (evaluation of losartan in the elderly study, ELITE). Lancet 1997;349:747–52.

[16] Pitt B, Poole-Wilson PA, Segal R, et al. Effect of losartan compared with captopril on mortality in patients with symptomatic heart failure: randomised trial–the Losartan Heart Failure Survival Study ELITE II [In Process Citation]. Lancet 2000;355:1582–7.

[17] Berlowitz MS, Latif F, Hankins SR, et al. Dose-dependent blockade of the angiotensin II type 1 receptor with losartan in normal volunteers. J Cardiovasc Pharmacol 2001;37:692–6.

[18] Granger CB, McMurray JJ, Yusuf S, et al. Effects of candesartan in patients with chronic heart failure and reduced left-ventricular systolic function intolerant to angiotensin-converting-enzyme inhibitors: the CHARM-Alternative trial. Lancet 2003;362:772–6.

[19] The SOLVD Investigators. Effect of enalapril on survival in patients with reduced left ventricular ejection fractions and congestive heart failure. N Engl J Med 1991;325:293–302.

[20] Flather MD, Yusuf S, Kober L, et al. Long-term ACE-inhibitor therapy in patients with heart failure or left-ventricular dysfunction: a systematic overview of data from individual patients. ACE-Inhibitor

Myocardial Infarction Collaborative Group [In Process Citation]. Lancet 2000;355:1575–81.

[21] Cohn JN, Tognoni G. A randomized trial of the angiotensin-receptor blocker valsartan in chronic heart failure. N Engl J Med 2001;345:1667–75.

[22] McMurray JJ, Ostergren J, Swedberg K, et al. Effects of candesartan in patients with chronic heart failure and reduced left-ventricular systolic function taking angiotensin-converting-enzyme inhibitors: the CHARM-Added trial. Lancet 2003;362:767–71.

[23] Hunt SA. ACC/AHA 2005 guideline update for the diagnosis and management of chronic heart failure in the adult: a report of the American College of Cardiology/American Heart Association Task Force on Practice Guidelines (Writing Committee to Update the 2001 Guidelines for the Evaluation and Management of Heart Failure). J Am Coll Cardiol 2005;46: e1–82.

[24] Dickstein K, Kjekshus J. Effects of losartan and captopril on mortality and morbidity in high-risk patients after acute myocardial infarction: the OPTIMAAL randomised trial. Optimal Trial in Myocardial Infarction with Angiotensin II Antagonist Losartan. Lancet 2002;360:752–60.

[25] Brenner BM, Cooper ME, de Zeeuw D, et al. Effects of losartan on renal and cardiovascular outcomes in patients with type 2 diabetes and nephropathy 10. N Engl J Med 2001;345:861–9.

[26] Dahlof B, Devereux RB, Kjeldsen SE, et al. Cardiovascular morbidity and mortality in the Losartan Intervention For Endpoint reduction in hypertension study (LIFE): a randomised trial against atenolol. Lancet 2002;359:995–1003.

[27] Pfeffer MA, McMurray JJ, Velazquez EJ, et al. Valsartan, captopril, or both in myocardial infarction complicated by heart failure, left ventricular dysfunction, or both. N Engl J Med 2003;349:1893–906.

[28] VALIANT: Implications and explanations 12931. HeartWire News. Available at: http://www.theheart.org/viewEntityDispatcherAction.do?primaryKey=470958. Accessed May 2007.

[29] Messerli FH, Re RN. Do we need yet another blocker of the renin-angiotensin system? J Am Coll Cardiol 2007;49:1164–5.

[30] Pitt B, Zannad F, Remme WJ, et al. The effect of spironolactone on morbidity and mortality in patients with severe heart failure. Randomized Aldactone Evaluation Study Investigators. N Engl J Med 1999;341:709–17.

[31] McKelvie RS, Yusuf S, Pericak D, et al. Comparison of candesartan, enalapril, and their combination in congestive heart failure: Randomized Evaluation of Strategies for Left Ventricular Dysfunction (RESOLVD) Pilot Study: The RESOLVD Pilot Study Investigators. Circulation 1999;100: 1056–64.

[32] Hunt SA, Abraham WT, Chin MH, et al. ACC/AHA 2005 Guideline Update for the Diagnosis and Management of Chronic Heart Failure in the Adult: a report of the American College of Cardiology/American Heart Association Task Force on Practice Guidelines (Writing Committee to Update the 2001 Guidelines for the Evaluation and Management of Heart Failure): developed in collaboration with the American College of Chest Physicians and the International Society for Heart and Lung Transplantation: endorsed by the Heart Rhythm Society. Circulation 2005;112:e154–235.

[33] Oh BH, Mitchell J, Herron JR, et al. Aliskiren, an oral renin inhibitor, provides dose-dependent efficacy and sustained 24-hour blood pressure control in patients with hypertension. J Am Coll Cardiol 2007;49:1157–63.

[34] O'Brien E, Barton J, Nussberger J, et al. Aliskiren reduces blood pressure and suppresses plasma renin activity in combination with a thiazide diuretic, an angiotensin-converting enzyme inhibitor, or an angiotensin receptor blocker. Hypertension 2007;49: 276–84.

[35] Mann DL, Deswal A, Bozkurt B, et al. New therapeutics for chronic heart failure. Annu Rev Med 2002;53:59–74.

ELSEVIER
SAUNDERS

Cardiol Clin 25 (2007) 581–594

CARDIOLOGY
CLINICS

Beta Blockers or Angiotensin-Converting-Enzyme Inhibitor/Angiotensin Receptor Blocker: What Should Be First?

Willem J. Remme, MD, PhD

Sticares Cardiovascular Research Institute, Rhoon, The Netherlands

During the last decades, appropriate drug therapy for heart failure has been well established. On the basis of unequivocal beneficial findings in large controlled studies, current international guidelines for the treatment of chronic heart failure advocate the use of angiotensin-converting-enzyme inhibitors (ACEI), beta blockers, aldosterone antagonists, and angiotensin receptor blockers (ARBs) as mandatory treatment to improve survival and/or clinical well-being in heart failure [1,2]. The rationale for the use of these neurohormonal antagonists is supported by their effect on cardiac remodeling, widely believed to be the pivotal mechanism leading to cardiac dysfunction and (worsening) heart failure, and contributing to various structural and functional changes instrumental in remodeling, such as apoptosis, hypertrophy, and cardiac fibrosis.

Overactivation of the renin-angiotensin and sympathetic systems, and increased aldosterone synthesis, mainly in target organs such as the heart, are major players in the remodeling process. Of these, activation of the sympathetic system is an early event, possibly preceding that of the renin-angiotensin system (RAS) [3]. In patients with left ventricular (LV) dysfunction, measurements of circulating neurohormones indicate an earlier rise in sympathetic nervous system activity than in that of the RAS. The temporal sequences of activation of these different neurohormonal systems and their timely blockade are the key to achieve optimal heart failure therapy.

It would appear logical, therefore, that the choice of which drug to use first, and when to follow up with subsequent other agents, would depend on recognition of these temporal sequences. As the sympathetic system appears to become activated before the RAS, it would seem logical to start with beta blockade before an RAS blocker (eg, an ACEI). Unfortunately, this is not the case.

The choice and timing of first and subsequent therapies in heart failure are determined by historical observations (first studies to be performed) on the one hand, and the stage of heart failure in which the respective drugs were tested and proven to be beneficial on the other.

As guidelines are by necessity based on strict evidence from these studies, they will invariably advocate initiation and timing of the various approved medications on the basis of this evidence. And as there are no data to contradict or question these decisions, they may be in error and patients are withheld more appropriate therapy, at least for some (precious) time.

Probably the most important and interesting question in this respect concerns the use of beta blockade versus ACE inhibition as first-line therapy for heart failure.

Angiotensin-converting-enzyme inhibition as first-line therapy in heart failure—a concept based on historical grounds

ACE inhibition has been recognized as a valuable treatment of chronic heart failure for two decades, well before the efficacy of the other

E-mail address: w.j.remme@sticares.org

neurohormonal antagonists became known. Pivotal studies, including Consensus I, Studies of Left Ventricular Dysfunction (SOLVD) treatment, and V-HeFT II, have clearly demonstrated the beneficial impact of these agents on mortality and worsening heart failure in patients with mild, moderate, or severe chronic heart failure [4–6]. Moreover, the SOLVD prevention study found that ACE inhibition could prevent the occurrence of symptomatic heart failure in patients with asymptomatic LV dysfunction [7]. In a slightly different population, patients with asymptomatic LV dysfunction or heart failure post-myocardial infarction (MI), various ACEI were found to improve survival and reduce the occurrence of (worsening) heart failure, resulting in fewer hospitalizations for cardiovascular reasons [8–10]. Importantly, side effects, including renal dysfunction and hyperkalemia, were relatively few in these study populations, which were often thoroughly selected to prevent the inclusion of elderly patients or those with significant renal dysfunction or low blood pressures.

As a consequence, ACEI have been considered the cornerstone of heart failure therapy for many years, as first-line treatment and applicable in all stages of heart failure, including asymptomatic LV dysfunction. Guidelines indicate that they should be used with or without diuretics as first-line therapy before treatment with other neurohormonal antagonists, notably beta blockade. This choice is, however, based on historical grounds: ACEI were the first drugs to be evaluated in long-term, controlled studies in patients who, up until then, were treated only with diuretics and/or digitalis glycosides. These studies were performed at a time when little or no knowledge existed about the usefulness of other neurohormonal antagonists in heart failure. In fact, in the early days of ACEI studies, the concept of neurohormonal activation being at the core of heart failure and the underlying remodeling process was hardly recognized. Initially, in the 1980s, ACEI were considered a special form of vasodilator, which by inhibiting the (by then) well-known vasoconstrictor effect of angiotensin II, could result in vasodilation and hemodynamic improvement in heart failure patients [11]. The cardiac anti-remodeling properties of ACEI (and of other neurohormonal antagonists) were scarcely known at that time. In a situation in which heart failure therapy focused on hemodynamic improvement, including positive inotropic therapy and unloading of the heart with vasodilatation, it was unthinkable to consider beta blockade for the treatment of heart failure—certainly not as a first choice.

Beta blockers were known for their negative inotropic properties and could lead to vasoconstriction during acute administration. However, had their efficacy in reducing cardiovascular hospitalizations—including those for heart failure—and decreasing death rates been known in those early days and the reasons behind it, it might have been a different story. Beta blockers could well have become the cornerstone of heart failure therapy and, possibly, the first drugs to consider in view of the early activation of the sympathoadrenergic system in this disease, before that of the RAS [3].

Unfortunately, it took a full decade before the results of the large, controlled beta blocker studies became available. And these results proved beyond a doubt the major beneficial effect of these agents on morbidity and mortality of the heart failure patient when administered long term.

These studies included the United States carvedilol trial [12], the Cardiac Insufficiency Bisoprolol Study (CIBIS) II [13], and MERIT-HF [14], with carvedilol, bisoprolol, and metoprolol succinate, respectively, performed in patients with mild to moderate heart failure; Copernicus [15], with carvedilol in patients with severe but stable heart failure; and Capricorn [16], with carvedilol in post-MI and LV dysfunction.

In all of these studies, a significant survival benefit was observed and, in most cases, a reduction in hospitalizations or for other cardiovascular reasons. More recently, the SENIORS study found a similar benefit for nebivolol in elderly heart failure patients [17].

In all these placebo-controlled studies, the beta blocker was given in addition to ACE inhibition; consequently, its indication became that of a second-line drug, to be started some time after initiation of ACE inhibition. How long that "some time" needs to be in a patient with manifest heart failure, those studies are unable to say, and current guidelines are not clear in this respect. Judging from the slow uptake of beta blockade per se in clinical practice, it may be quite a while for patients to receive this mandatory treatment, if they receive it at all [18].

This situation poses two questions: (1) Should ACE inhibition always be first-line therapy, or could beta blockade replace ACE inhibition in this respect? (2) Is it necessary to combine the two types of drugs at an early stage or not?

Large, long-term clinical studies comparing both types of drugs head-to-head may be required to answer the first question, which inevitably will raise questions regarding ethics and costs.

To answer the second question would require a complex set of studies with different timing intervals between the two drugs and, again, a large patient population. Obviously, studies with surrogate endpoints needing fewer patients and shorter time spans are required. One such surrogate endpoint is cardiac remodeling [19].

Why beta blockade may reverse cardiac remodeling

Various mechanisms contribute to cardiac remodeling, including mechanical stretch, activation of mechano-sensitive ion channels, neurohormonal activation, cytokine production, inflammation, inducible nitric oxide (NO) synthase activation, oxidative stress, apoptosis, and ischemia [20]. These factors often work in tandem and/or interrelate. Sympathetic (over) activation, but also angiotensin II, affects cytokine production, including TNFα, which increases inducible NO, leading to excess NO and, subsequently, to oxidative stress and apoptosis [21,22]. Mechanical stretch, important in the remodeling process, activates angiotensin II and the α1-adrenergic system, among others [23]. Thus, both blockers of the RAS and beta blockers could be useful in modulating cardiac remodeling.

Why then beta blockade specifically?

First, as mentioned, activation of the sympathetic system occurs early after cardiac injury, leading to heart failure, possibly earlier than that of the RAS.

Second, there is a high cardiac sympathetic tone in heart failure, resulting in local levels of norepinephrine high enough to become toxic for the cardiomyocyte [24] and to lead to catecholamine-induced necrosis and cardiomyocyte apoptosis [25]. Beta blockade as well as desensitization of beta receptors may counteract these untoward effects [26]. Also, beta blockade has been shown to reduce pro-apoptotic factors, such as Bax, and to increase anti-apoptotic factors, including Bcl-2 and Bcl X (S), altering the balance of these factors in a favorable anti-apoptotic way [27]. In this process, antioxidant properties play an important role [28]. Carvedilol reduces oxidative stress-induced apoptosis, in contrast to metoprolol, atenolol, propanolol, or

a combination of alpha and beta blockade [29]. In contrast, the effect of a combination of the antioxidant N-acetyl-L-cysteine and propranolol was comparable to that of carvedilol, suggesting a selective antioxidative role of carvedilol. Moreover, whereas beta blockade up-regulates reduced SERCA levels post- MI, and improves impaired cardiac function and remodeling under these conditions, these effects were more pronounced with carvedilol than with metoprolol [30].

Heart rate reduction is a further mechanism that may be involved in reversing the remodeling process with beta blockade. The inherent longer diastolic period allows for longer coronary perfusion, whereas the reduction in heart rate impacts on myocardial oxygen demand. As a consequence, myocardial ischemia may be less during beta blocker therapy. Subclinical ischemia and hibernating myocardium may be important mechanisms that contribute to impaired cardiac function following an MI, and can be significantly reduced during long-term therapy with carvedilol [31].

A further possible argument to expect an effect of beta blockade on remodeling relates to cardiac metabolism. Sympathetic activation in heart failure shifts energy production from carbohydrate to free fatty acid use (enhanced lipolysis). This means less high-energy phosphate (ATP) production for the same amount of available oxygen. Beta blockade reverses the process and increases the dependency on carbohydrates, thus improving the efficiency of the energy-production process with more ATP available for cardiac contraction.

Together, there are ample reasons to expect beta blockers to ameliorate cardiac remodeling. However, are the different beta blocking agents that are currently accepted in the treatment of heart failure comparable in this respect?

Cardiac remodeling: does it matter which beta blocker?

Of the beta blocking agents approved for heart failure treatment in current guidelines, only metoprolol and carvedilol have been studied and compared in a sizeable number of studies in regard to their effect on cardiac remodeling. Metoprolol is a selective beta-1 adrenergic antagonist, whereas carvedilol has beta-1, beta-2, and alpha-1 receptor-blocking properties.

All three adrenergic receptors are linked to downstream cellular signaling pathways leading to molecular signals for remodeling, albeit through different pathways. This is important as blockade of one receptor would leave remodeling to continue through the others. As such, it makes sense to block all three to derive most of the effect of the beta blocker. Myocardial stretch increases alpha-adrenergic activation, which leads to cardiac hypertrophy and myocardial toxicity. In addition, alpha-1 activation results in coronary and peripheral (renal) vasoconstriction, potentially increasing the risk of myocardial ischemia and other cardiovascular and cardiorenal complications in heart failure. In the COMET study, carvedilol, when compared with metoprolol tartrate, significantly reduced the occurrence of cardiovascular death, stroke death, nonfatal MIs, and unstable angina [32].

Beta-2 receptor activation diminishes the occurrence of apoptosis. However, this potential beneficial effect may be offset by the facilitation of norepinephrine release through presynaptic cardiac beta-2 receptors, which are percentage-wise increased in heart failure. Also, beta-2 receptor stimulation may activate myocardial fibrosis, and may be arrhythmogenic [33,34].

Nevertheless, of the three adrenergic receptors, the beta-1 is probably the most important in the remodeling process. For instance, pro-apoptotic factors, such as Bcl-X(s) expression, increase through beta-1 receptor stimulation, and beta-1 antagonists (eg, atenolol and metoprolol-l) can reduce cardiomyocyte apoptosis post-MI mainly through the increase of anti-apoptotic Bcl-2 expression and Bcl-2/Bax ratio.

Would this then favor specific beta-1 antagonists? Not necessarily, as carvedilol, in comparison with the beta-1 selective agent metoprolol, has a tighter binding to the beta-1 receptor and, hence, a longer-lasting blocking effect [35]. Moreover, carvedilol has been shown to exert more potent anti-adrenergic effects than metoprolol in heart failure [36].

Together, these arguments would favor carvedilol to metoprolol when it comes to reversing remodeling. Indeed, several studies comparing the two beta blockers in regard to their effect on remodeling indicate a more pronounced inhibiting effect of carvedilol. Sanderson and colleagues [37] observed a greater decrease in LV volumes with carvedilol than metoprolol in heart failure patients, whereas Metra and colleagues [38] found a significantly greater increase in LV ejection fraction with carvedilol after approximately 1 year of treatment. The latter was also shown

in a meta-analysis encompassing all available controlled studies with the two compounds [39]. Finally, the COMET study unequivocally demonstrated a significantly better effect of carvedilol on survival and hospitalizations for cardiovascular reasons, including heart failure, compared with metoprolol in chronic heart failure patients [40].

Why beta blockers first may lead to improved survival and better quality of life compared with inhibitors of the renin-angiotensin system

As mentioned, activation of the sympathetic system precedes that of the RAS in heart failure and is one of underlying mechanisms for subsequent RAS stimulation [3]. Pretreatment with a beta blocker prevents "ACEI escape" and contributes to a greater suppressing effect of ACEI on angiotensin II production.

Increased renal sympathetic drive promotes salt and water retention; beta blockade may prevent this [41]. Also, it may decrease untoward increases in serum creatinine during ACEI therapy, thereby preventing cardiorenal complications [42].

Finally, in contrast to ACE inhibition, beta blockade results in a significant inhibition of ventricular tachy-arrhythmias and reduction of sudden death [14,43,44]. The latter is particularly important in mild to moderate heart failure, where a first-line drug will be typically prescribed. Sudden cardiac death is more prominent as mode of death in these early stages than in more advanced heart failure.

Renin-angiotensin system inhibition or beta blockade: which is the better anti-remodeling agent?

Are there reasons to believe that RAS inhibition would better protect against remodeling than would beta blockade, especially carvedilol? Arguments in favor of RAS inhibition include the more extensive anti-RAS activity, a greater hypotensive effect (particularly with ARBs), and, in case of ACE inhibition—and to a lesser extent the ARBs—increased bradykinin and NO production.

Arguments in favor of beta blockade include the comprehensive adrenergic blockade with cardiac and renal anti-adrenergic effects; a greater anti-ischemic profile; heart rate reduction; and probably more extensive antioxidative, anti-endothelin, and anti-apoptotic effects. This larger scale of mechanisms through which to affect remodeling, and, hence, heart failure progression would appear to favor beta blockade. Are the results of controlled clinical studies in line with this suggestion?

Available ACEI trials in heart failure indicate a clear effect on progression of remodeling. The SOLVD echo substudy compared enalapril with placebo over a 1-year treatment period. Although placebo-treated patients continued to increase their cardiac volumes, enalapril-treated patients did not (Fig. 1) [45]. In a different context, post-MI LV dysfunction, captopril had a similar effect on cardiac volumes during 2 years of follow-up [46], whereas in the PREAMI study, in elderly patients with a normal cardiac function post-MI, perindopril also prevented the increase in LV volumes observed in placebo-treated patients [47]. Of importance, whereas the older studies were not in addition to beta blockade, the PREAMI study was. Also, in the VaL-HeFT echocardiographic study, the ARB valsartan was administered in addition to ACEI and/or beta blockade [48].

In none of these studies (except for VaL-HeFT) did therapy result in a reversal of remodeling (ie, in cardiac volumes becoming smaller over time).

This finding contrasts with the observations from beta blocker trials. In the Australia and New Zealand study in patients with mild heart failure

and LV dysfunction, carvedilol significantly reduced LV volumes compared with placebo [49]. In the CAPRICORN trial in patients with LV dysfunction post-MI, carvedilol also reduced cardiac volumes over a 6-month period [50].

The problem in interpreting these studies as to the anti-remodeling effect of the beta blocker is that carvedilol was added to pre-existing therapy with ACEI in most patients. The combination of two anti-remodeling therapies may well have resulted in reversal of remodeling with a decrease in cardiac volumes, which may not necessarily occur with either drug alone.

To answer the question of whether beta blockade provides better protection against cardiac remodeling than does ACE inhibition requires a head-to-head comparison between the two drug regimens over a prolonged period of time. At present, two such studies are available.

Head-to-head comparison between angiotensin-converting-enzyme inhibition and beta blockade on cardiac remodeling

Sliwa and colleagues [51] compared carvedilol and perindopril in a single-center, nonblinded study in 78 patients with New York Heart Association (NYHA) class II/III heart failure due to idiopathic-dilated cardiomyopathy and LV dysfunction. Patients received either perindopril in

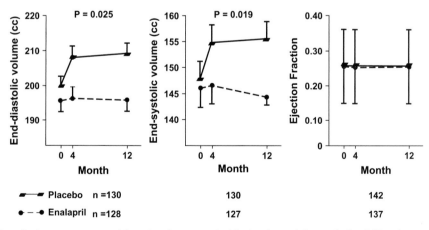

Fig. 1. Effect of a 1-year treatment with enalapril compared with placebo on left ventricular (LV) volumes and ejection fraction in the SOLVD echocardiographic substudy in patients with LV dysfunction from both the treatment and prevention arms of SOLVD. Enalapril significantly prevents the increase in end-diastolic and end-systolic volumes observed in the placebo group. (*Data from* Greenberg B, Quinones MA, Koilpillai C, et al. Effects of long-term enalapril therapy on cardiac structure and function in patients with left ventricular dysfunction. Results of the SOLVD echocardiographic study. Circulation 1995;91:2573–81.)

a target dose of 8 mg or carvedilol, up-titrated to 25 mg twice a day for 6 months. After that period, the comparator drug was added to the initial treatment for another period of 6 months.

In the carvedilol group, LV ejection fraction increased by 11% more than in the perindopril group, a difference that was already significant after the monotherapy period at 6 months (Fig. 2). Also, at 12 months both LV end-systolic and end-diastolic dimensions had decreased in the carvedilol-first group, compared with baseline. In the ACEI patients this did not happen, but, comparable to the experience in the SOLVD study,

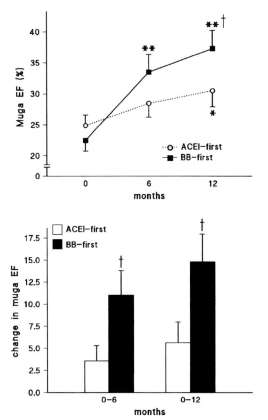

Fig. 2. Impact of initiating carvedilol before perindopril therapy (beta blocker [BB]–first group) compared with the effect of the commencement of perindopril first (ACEI–first group) on LV ejection fraction (EF), determined using radionuclide techniques. Carvedilol results in a significantly greater increase in LV EF after 6 months of monotherapy, which pertains during subsequent combined BB/ACEI treatment. (*From* Sliwa K, Norton GR, Kone N, et al. Impact of initiating carvedilol before angiotensin converting enzyme inhibitor therapy on cardiac function in newly diagnosed heart failure. J Am Coll Cardiol 2004;44:1825–30; with permission.)

ventricular dimensions did not change. The better anti-remodeling effect of carvedilol resulted in a significant reduction in plasma NT-proBNP levels, whereas these did not change in the perindopril patients (Fig. 3). Moreover, at 12 months there was a significantly greater benefit in terms of NYHA classification in the carvedilol-first as compared with the perindopril-first group. The limitations of this study are the small sample size, open-label design, and, particularly, the short duration of the monotherapy period. By contrast, the second study comparing ACE inhibition with beta blockade on remodeling, the CArvedilol Remodeling in Mild heart failure EvaluatioN (CARMEN), was significantly longer.

CArvedilol Remodeling in Mild heart failure EvaluatioN study

The CARMEN study evaluated patients with NYHA class II/III heart failure and LV dysfunction due to ischemic heart disease (approximately 50% had a previous MI), hypertension (approximately 30%), idiopathic-dilated cardiomyopathy, and valvular disease [52]. Patients had to be clinically stable for 2 weeks before entry, during which time ACE inhibition (present in two thirds of the study population) was withdrawn. The aim was to evaluate whether carvedilol alone would better prevent against remodeling than ACE inhibition with enalapril. Moreover, the effect of both monotherapies was compared with that of their combination. For the treatments to fully develop their effect on remodeling, a long (18 months) double-blind treatment period was chosen. Patients were randomized to enalapril alone (10 mg twice daily), carvedilol alone (25 mg twice daily), or the combination of these regimens. This necessitated a complicated, double-blind titration scheme, in which in the combination arm carvedilol was titrated first, followed by enalapril, and in the monotherapy groups placebo was added during the second titration period. The primary and secondary endpoints concerned the changes in LV end-systolic index (measured at an echo corelab) at 6, 12, and 18 months of double-blind treatment between and within the groups.

The results of CARMEN, performed on 572 patients, unequivocally indicate that the combination therapy (with carvedilol up-titrated first) provided a better anti-remodeling effect than enalapril alone (Fig. 4) [53]. The difference between the combination arm and carvedilol alone was also in favor of combination therapy, but

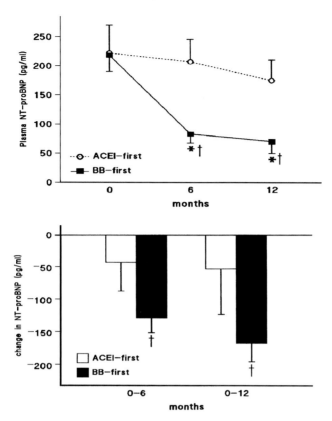

Fig. 3. Impact of initiating carvedilol before perindopril therapy (BB–first group) compared with the effect of the commencement of perindopril first (ACEI–first group) on plasma N-terminal-pro-brain natriuretic peptide (NT-pro-BNP) concentrations. Carvedilol reduces NT-pro-BNP already after 6 months of monotherapy in contrast to perindopril. (*From* Sliwa K, Norton GR, Kone N, et al. Impact of initiating carvedilol before angiotensin converting enzyme inhibitor therapy on cardiac function in newly diagnosed heart failure. J Am Coll Cardiol 2004;44:1825–30; with permission.)

smaller than in the enalapril comparison. Of importance, carvedilol alone significantly decreased end-systolic volumes compared with baseline, whereas no changes occurred in the enalapril-alone arm (Fig. 5). Similar directional findings as in LV end-systolic volumes were observed in end-diastolic volumes and ejection fraction.

In this mild heart failure study (62%–68% in the three arms were NYHA class II), serious adverse events were few (28% of patients in the combined-treatment arm, 29% in carvedilol-alone arm, and 34% in the enalapril-alone arm). Also, the number of withdrawals during up-titration and maintenance therapy was comparable between groups, varying between 18% (combination and carvedilol arms) and 21% (enalapril alone). There was no difference in survival rates. Also, cardiovascular hospitalizations and hospitalizations for heart failure were comparable

despite a tendency toward a higher incidence with enalapril.

These results from CARMEN suggest that both in terms of efficacy and safety, beta blockade alone is not inferior to ACE inhibition, and may even be better—a suggestion that is supported by the findings of Sliwa and colleagues [51].

However, these studies focused on remodeling, a reliable structural surrogate for the progression of the heart failure syndrome [19], but not large enough to provide sufficient mortality and morbidity endpoints. That was the aim of the CIBIS III trial.

Cardiac Insufficiency Bisoprolol Study III

The CIBIS II study was designed to assess noninferiority of beta blockade first with bisoprolol to ACE inhibition first (enalapril), followed by

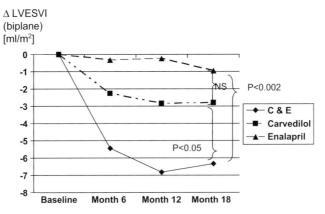

Fig. 4. Mean change from baseline in left ventricular end–systolic volume index (LVE–SVI) in the intention-to-treat (ITT) population. In the combination arm, LVE–SVI is significantly more reduced than in both monotherapy arms, during the entire course of the study. Differences between groups, P values valid for comparisons at all time points. C, carvedilol; E, enalapril. (*From* Remme WJ, Riegger G, Hildebrandt P, et al, on behalf of the CARMEN investigators. The benefits of early combination treatment of carvedilol and an ACE-inhibitor in mild heart failure and left ventricular systolic dysfunction. The Carvedilol and Ace-inhibitor Remodeling Mild heart failure EvaluatioN trial (CARMEN). Cardiovasc Drugs Ther 2004;18:57–66; with permission).

combination of both therapies on a combined endpoint of all-cause death and all-cause hospitalizations in patients with mild to moderate heart failure and LV dysfunction [54]. To this end, 1010 patients, 72.5 years of age, were up-titrated to maximally 10-mg bisoprolol once daily or to 10 mg twice daily in a randomized, open-label (unblinded) design and continued monotherapy for 6 months, followed by a combined treatment period, which lasted between 6 and 24 months, and included the second up-titration phase. As

the monotherapy phase did include the first up-titration period, which lasted approximately 2.5 months, this left only 3.5 months for the maintenance period during which bisoprolol alone was administered at the best tolerated dose. The respective time intervals for enalapril-treated patients were 1 and 5 months, respectively. Hence, the maximum maintenance period on bisoprolol alone was 16 weeks, on enalapril alone 22 weeks.

Although the Kaplan-Meier plots shown in Fig. 6 clearly suggests the two treatments to be

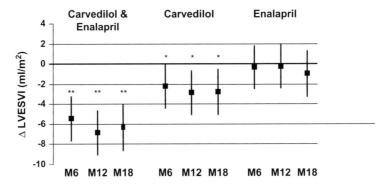

Fig. 5. Mean change from baseline in LVE–SVI in the ITT population. Both the combination and carvedilol treatment arms show a significant reduction in LVE–SVI from baseline. No changes occur in the enalapril-alone arm. Bars represent 95% confidence intervals. P values for within-group changes are depicted (**$P < .01$, *$P < .05$). M, month; for further abbreviations see Fig 4. (*From* Remme WJ, Riegger G, Hildebrandt P, et al, on behalf of the CARMEN investigators. The benefits of early combination treatment of carvedilol and an ACE-inhibitor in mild heart failure and left ventricular systolic dysfunction. The Carvedilol and Ace-inhibitor Remodeling Mild heart failure EvaluatioN trial (CARMEN). Cardiovasc Drugs Ther 2004;18:57–66; with permission).

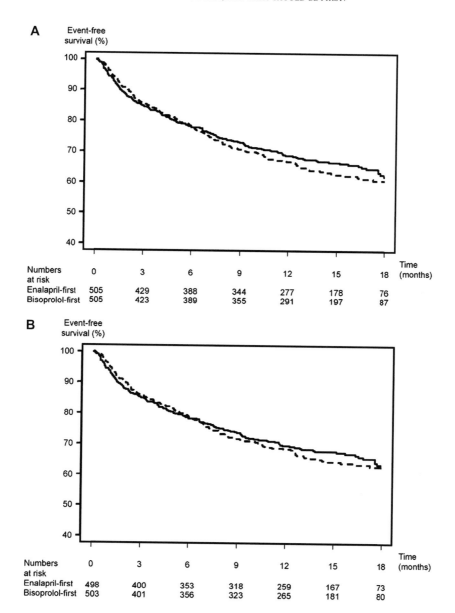

Fig. 6. Kaplan-Meier plots of the combined primary endpoint (all-cause death or all-cause hospitalization) in the ITT sample (*A*) and in the per-protocol sample (*B*) in CIBIS III. The bisoprolol-first group is indicated by the solid line, the enalapril-first group by the dotted line. The curves suggest a comparable effect of bisoprolol-first and enalapril-first. However, the prespecified criteria for noninferiority for bisoprolol in the per-protocol analysis (primary efficacy variable) were not met ($P = .046$, significance set at $P = .025$). (*From* Willenheimer R, van Veldhuisen DJ, Silke B, et al, on behalf of the CIBIS III investigators. Effect on survival and hospitalization of initiating treatment for chronic heart failure with bisoprolol followed by enalapril, as compared with the opposite sequence. Results of the Randomized Cardiac Insufficiency Bisoprolol study (CIBIS) III. Circulation 2005;112:2426–35; with permission.)

equal, the primary endpoint (non-inferiority in the per-protocol analysis) was not met, and the trial also did not meet criteria for superiority of biso-prolol-first treatment [55].

Similar numbers of patients were withdrawn during the study, and although adverse event and serious adverse event rates were comparable during the entire study period, there were more serious event reports during the bisoprolol-only phase as compared with the enalapril-only arm. Also, there was a tendency for bisoprolol to result in more worsening heart failure requiring hospi-talization or occurring while in hospital (63 versus 51 enalapril patients, hazard ratio [HR] 1.25, 95% CI, 0.87—1.81, $P = .23$ (Fig. 7).

Of importance, only 65% of bisoprolol-first patients received the target dose of 10 mg, compared with 84% in the enalapril-first arm. Also, at the end of the study, 53% took target doses of bisoprolol in the enalapril-first group. These relatively low percentages may well be the result of the unblinded study design, but also

could reflect the response to a selective beta-1 antagonist without vasodilating properties, such as carvedilol.

Another concern with CIBIS III relates to the study design in which a long combined treatment phase was preceded by a relatively short period of monotherapy. Although the aim was to compare beta blockade and ACE inhibition head-to-head, this was done during short and (at least where target doses are concerned) unequal study periods between the two groups (maximum 16 weeks for bisoprolol versus maximum 22 weeks for enalap-ril). It is questionable whether any drug-specific effect would have had enough time to develop a meaningful difference between the two regimens. Nevertheless, the results of the 6-month mono-therapy phase should be published to (hopefully) get a meaningful idea of the study [56]. As it now stands, the relative long period of combined treat-ment will most likely produce similar results in both groups (and has done so), and "drown" any effect of either drug alone.

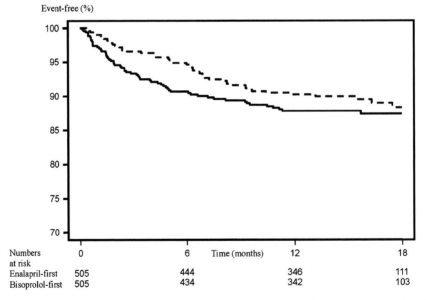

Fig. 7. Kaplan-Meier plot of patients with worsening heart failure requiring hospitalization or occurring while in hos-pital in the ITT sample (CIBIS III). The bisoprolol-first group is indicated by the solid line, the enalapril-first group by the dotted line. A tendency was seen for more patients with worsening heart failure after 6 months in the bisoprolol-only group, although the difference during the entire study is not significant (HR 1.25, 95% CI, 0.87–1.81, $P = .23$). (*From* Willenheimer R, van Veldhuisen DJ, Silke B, et al, on behalf of the CIBIS III investigators. Effect on survival and hos-pitalization of initiating treatment for chronic heart failure with bisoprolol followed by enalapril, as compared with the opposite sequence. Results of the Randomized Cardiac Insufficiency Bisoprolol study (CIBIS) III. Circulation 2005;112:2426–35; with permission.)

What is the message to take home from these studies?

For the reasons provided above, it is difficult to take home a message from CIBIS III. Can one suggest that, with an interval of several months between starting either a beta blocker or an ACEI and then adding the other treatment, patients are optimally (although possibly comparably) treated? One cannot, as the study was not designed for that—a third arm including a combined-treatment arm as in CARMEN, not being available.

On the contrary, the results of CARMEN indicate that early combined treatment provides a better result than giving either drug alone for any given time (the difference was already significant at 6-month treatment).

Does CIBIS III suggest that beta blockade with bisoprolol as first-line therapy is superior or non-inferior to ACE inhibition as first-line treatment? It does not, not only as (formally) the primary endpoint was not reached—let alone superiority of bisoprolol proven—but rather as information is not available regarding the actual period during which the drugs were compared head-to-head. Moreover, it is uncertain whether the relatively short period of the latter would allow a relevant comparison. Beta blockade requires several months to achieve maximum change in LV remodeling [57], and the 16-week maximum period for patients to be on bisoprolol monotherapy may not have been enough.

Which messages can be taken home from the CArvedilol Remodeling in Mild heart failure EvaluatioN study

The first message is that treatment with beta blockade should not be delayed in heart failure, but should be combined with ACE inhibition at an early stage. The majority of patients in the CARMEN study had mild heart failure, and in those patients the combination (one drug up-titrated immediately after the other) led to a greater reduction of cardiac remodeling than either drug alone. One may expect this to lead to a greater retardation of heart failure progression.

This is an important message, as guidelines do not stress this. And in clinical practice beta blockers are grossly underused, despite the well-known fact that when beta blockers are added to ACEI, remodeling is not only reversed, but also in

an approximately 35%, mortality is reduced and clinical well-being is improved significantly.

Also, beta blockers (and ACEI as well) are prescribed in low dosages, well under the target level used in the controlled studies. Moreover, there may be an extended period of time before patients receive the second drug after ACE inhibition, usually the beta blocker. In clinical practice, up-titration of the second drug invariably occurs to a lower dose level than when given as a first-line drug (as shown in CIBIS III), which also reflects the reluctance of the clinician toward a more aggressive approach in heart failure, particularly in the milder forms.

It is crucial therefore that clinicians understand the rationale and need of multiple, simultaneous neurohormonal antagonists at all stages of heart failure (aldosterone antagonists possibly entering the stage also in the milder heart failure patient).

The second message from the CARMEN study is that carvedilol is at least as, or possibly more, effective than ACE inhibition in reversing remodeling. Although in the comparison between the two drugs the difference in favor of carvedilol was not significant, it was so at earlier time points during the study. Also, carvedilol—and not enalapril—significantly reduced cardiac volumes from baseline. That approximately two thirds of the population had been treated before is unlikely to matter here, as in the other patients enalapril also did not result in significant volume changes [58]. Of importance in both the combined and carvedilol-alone arm, up-titration of carvedilol first was very well tolerated and did not lead to more adverse events or drop-outs from the study than in the enalapril-alone arm.

The potentially better effect on remodeling by carvedilol, the excellent safety aspects during the study and tolerability of carvedilol during up-titration before the introduction of ACE inhibition in CARMEN, suggests a role for beta blockade as first-line therapy in heart failure and ACE inhibition as second choice. Whether this holds for all patients is unclear. Obviously, patients who are unstable and have clear signs of rapidly worsening heart failure are not candidates for beta blockade first. Such patients need to be stabilized first with ACE inhibition or ARB and diuretics. However, stable patients with mild to moderate heart failure (such as those studied in CARMEN, in the study by Sliwa and colleagues, and in CIBIS III) might well be candidates for beta blockade as first-line therapy. This may be particularly true for those with a relatively fast heart rate [59]. As such, the results of CARMEN, the study by Sliwa and colleagues, and possibly CIBIS III indicate that the mandatory first-line treatment with ACEI needs to be reconsidered. Clinicians dealing with heart failure patients should not be forced to follow a dogmatic approach, but rather have the opportunity to choose the best order of treatment in the individual patient.

References

[1] Hunt SA, Abraham WT, Chin MH, et al. ACC/AHA 2005 guideline update for the diagnosis and management of chronic heart failure in the adult. Circulation 2005;112:e154–235.

[2] Swedberg K, Cleland J, Dargie H, et al. Guidelines for the diagnosis and treatment of chronic heart failure: executive summary (update 2005). Eur Heart J 2005;26:1115–40.

[3] Francis GS, Benedict C, Johnston DE, et al. Comparison of neuroendocrine activation in patients with left ventricular dysfunction with and without congestive heart failure: a substudy of the Studies Of Left Ventricular Dysfunction (SOLVD). Circulation 1990;82:1724–9.

[4] CONSENSUS Trial Study Group. Effect of enalapril on mortality in severe congestive heart failure. Results of the North Scandinavian enalapril survival study. N Engl J Med 1987;316:1429–35.

[5] The SOLVD Investigators. Effects of enalapril on survival in patients with reduced left ventricular ejection fractions and congestive heart failure. N Engl J Med 1991;325:293–302.

[6] Cohn JN, Johnson G, Ziesche S, et al. A comparison of enalapril with hydralazine-isosorbide dinitrate in the treatment of chronic congestive heart failure. N Engl J Med 1991;325:303–10.

[7] The SOLVD Investigators. Effects of enalapril on mortality and the development of heart failure in asymptomatic patients with reduced left ventricular ejection fractions. N Engl J Med 1992;327:685–91.

[8] Acute Infarction Ramipril Efficacy (AIRE) Investigators. Effects of ramipril on mortality and morbidity of survivors of acute myocardial infarction with clinical evidence of heart failure. Lancet 1993;342:821–8.

[9] Pfeffer MA, Braunwald E, Moyé LA, et al, on behalf of the SAVE investigators. Effect of captopril on mortality and morbidity in patients with left ventricular dysfunction after myocardial infarction. N Engl J Med 1992;327:669–77.

[10] Køber L, Torp-Pederson C, Carlsen JE, et al, for the TRACE Study Group. A clinical trial of the angiotensin-converting-enzyme inhibitor trandolapril in patients with left ventricular dysfunction after myocardial infarction. N Engl J Med 1995;333:1670–6.

[11] Remme WJ. Vasodilator therapy without converting enzyme inhibition in congestive heart failure– usefulness and limitations. Cardiovasc Drugs Ther 1989;3: 375–96.

[12] Packer M, Bristow MR, Cohn JN, et al. The effect of carvedilol on morbidity and mortality in patients with chronic heart failure. U.S. Carvedilol Heart Failure Study Group. N Engl J Med 1996;334: 1349–55.

[13] CIBIS II Investigators and Committees. The Cardiac Insufficiency Bisoprolol Study II (CIBIS II): a randomised trial. Lancet 1999;353:9–13.

[14] Hjalmarson A, Goldstein S, Fagerberg B, et al. Effect of metoprolol CR/XL in chronic heart failure: metoprolol CR/XL randomized intervention trial in congestive heart failure (MERIT-HF). Lancet 1999;353:2001–7.

[15] Packer M, Coats AJS, Fowler MB, et al, for the Carvedilol Prospective Randomized Cumulative Survival Study Group (COPERNICUS). Effect of carvedilol on survival in severe chronic heart failure. N Engl J Med 2001;344:1651–8.

[16] The CAPRICORN Investigators. Effect of carvedilol on outcome after myocardial infarction in patients with left ventricular dysfunction: the CAPRICORN randomised trial. Lancet 2001;357: 1385–90.

[17] Flather MD, Shibata MC, Coats AJ, et al. Randomized trial to determine the effect of nebivolol on mortality and cardiovascular hospital admission in elderly patients with heart failure (SENIORS). Eur Heart J 2005;26:215–25.

[18] Cleland JG, Cohen-Solal A, Cosin Aguilar J, et al. Management of heart failure in primary care (the IMPROVEMENT of Heart Failure Programme): an international survey. Lancet 2002; 360:1631–9.

[19] Cohn JN. Remodeling as an end-point in heart failure therapy. Cardiovasc Drugs Ther 2004;18:7–8.

[20] Remme WJ. Pharmacological modulation of cardiovascular remodeling: a guide to heart failure therapy. Cardiovasc Drugs Ther 2003;17:349–60.

[21] Ungureanu-Longrois D, Balligand JL, Simmons SW, et al. Induction of nitric oxide synthase activity by cytokines in ventricular myocytes is necessary but not sufficient to decrease contractile responsiveness to β-adrenergiec agonists. Circ Res 1995;77: 494–502.

[22] Li X, Moody MR, Engl D, et al. Cardiac-specific overexpression of tumor necrosis factor-α causes oxidative stress and contractile dysfunction in mouse diaphragm. Circulation 2000;102:1690–6.

[23] Yamazaki T, Komuro I, Kudoh S, et al. Role of ion channels and exchangers in mechanical stretch-induced cardiomyocyte hypertrophy. Circ Res 1998; 82:430–7.

[24] Mann DL, Kent RL, Parsons B, et al. Adrenergic effects on the biology of the adult mammalian cardiocyte. Circulation 1992;24:549–64.

[25] Communal C, Singh K, Pimentel DR, et al. Norepinephrine stimulates apoptosis in adult rat ventricular myocytes by activation of beta-adrenergic pathway. Circulation 1998;98:1329–34.

[26] Tan LB, Benjamin IJ, Clark WA. Beta-adrenergic receptor desensitization may serve a cardioprotective role. Cardiovasc Res 1992;26:608–14.

[27] Prabhu SD, Wang G, Luo J, et al. Beta-adrenergic receptor blockade modulates Bcl-X(S) expression and reduces apoptosis in failing myocardium. J Mol Cell Cardiol 2003;35:483–93.

[28] Kawai K, Qin F, Shite J, et al. Importance of antioxidant and antiapoptotic effects of beta-receptor blockers in heart failure therapy. Am J Physiol Heart Circ Physiol 2004;287:H1003–12.

[29] Wang R, Miura T, Harada N, et al. Pleiotropic effects of the beta-adrenoceptor blocker carvedilol on calcium regulation during oxidative stress-induced apoptosis in cardiomyocytes. J Pharmacol Exp Ther 2006;318:45–52.

[30] Sun YL, Hu SJ, Wang LH, et al. Effect of betablockers on cardiac function and calcium handling protein in postinfarction heart failure rats. Chest 2005;128:1812–21.

[31] Cleland JGF, Pennell DJ, Ray SG, et al. Myocardial viability as a determinant of the ejection fraction response to carvedilol in patients with heart failure (CHRISTMAS trial): randomised, controlled trial. Lancet 2003;362:14–21.

[32] Remme WJ, Torp-Pedersen C, Cleland JGF, et al. Carvedilol protects better against vascular events than metoprolol in heart failure: Results from COMET. J Am Coll Cardiol 2007;49:963–71.

[33] Du XJ, Autelitano D, Dilley RJ, et al. ß₂-adrenergic overexpression exacerbates development of heart failure after aortic stenosis. Circulation 2000;101: 71–7.

[34] Billman GE, Castillo LC, Hensley J, et al. ß₂-adrenergic receptor antagonists protect against ventricular fibrillation. In vivo and in vitro evidence for enhanced sensitivity to ß₂-adrenergic stimulation in animals susceptible to sudden death. Circulation 1997; 96:1914–22.

[35] Kindermann M, Maack C, Schaller S, et al. Carvedilol but not metoprolol reduces β-adrenergic responsiveness after complete elimination from plasma in vivo. Circulation 2004;109:3182–9.

[36] Kohno T, Yoshikawa T, Yoshizawa A, et al. Carvedilol exerts more potent antiadrenergics effect than metoprolol in heart failure. Cardiovasc Drugs Ther 2005;19:347–55.

[37] Sanderson JE, Chan SKW, Yip G, et al. Beta-blockade in heart failure. A comparison of carvedilol with metoprolol. J Am Coll Cardiol 1999;34:1522–8.

[38] Metra M, Gibbini R, Nodari S, et al. Differential effects of beta-blockers in patients with heart failure. A prospective, randomized, double-blind comparison of the long-term effects of metoprolol versus carvedilol. Circulation 2000;102:546–51.

[39] Packer M, Antonopoulos GV, Berlin JA, et al. Comparative effects of carvedilol and metoprolol on left ventricular ejection fraction in heart failure: results of a meta-analysis. Am Heart J 2001;141:899–907.

[40] Poole-Wilson PA, Swedberg K, Cleland JGF, et al. Comparison of carvedilol and metoprolol on clinical outcomes in patients with chronic heart failure. Results of the Carvedilol Or Metoprolol European Trial (COMET). Lancet 2003;362:7–13.

[41] Schrier RW, Abraham WT. Hormones and hemodynamics in heart failure. N Engl J Med 1999;341: 577–85.

[42] Knight EL, Glynn RJ, McIntyre KM, et al. Predictors of decreased renal function in patients with heart failure during angiotensin—converting enzyme inhibitor therapy: results from the studies of left ventricular dysfunction (SOLVD). Am Heart J 1999;138:849–55.

[43] Garg R, Yusuf S. Overview of randomized trials of angiotensin-converting enzyme inhibitors on mortality and morbidity in patients with heart failure. Collaborative Group on ACE Inhibitor Trials. JAMA 1995;273:1450–6.

[44] Remme WJ, Cleland JG, Erhardt L, et al. Effect of carvedilol and metoprolol on the mode of death in patients with heart failure. Eur J Heart Fail, in press.

[45] Greenberg B, Quinones MA, Koilpillai C, et al. Effects of long-term enalapril therapy on cardiac structure and function in patients with left ventricular dysfunction. Results of the SOLVD echocardiographic study. Circulation 1995;91:2573–81.

[46] St John Sutton M, Pfeffer MA, Moye L, et al. Cardiovascular death and left ventricular remodeling two years after myocardial infarction: baseline predictors and impact of long-term use of captopril: information from the Survival and Ventricular Enlargement (SAVE) trial. Circulation 1997;96:3294–9.

[47] The PREAMI Investigators. Effects of angiotensinconverting enzyme inhibition with perindopril on left ventricular remodelling and clinical outcome. Arch Intern Med 2006;166:659–66.

[48] Wong M, Staszewsky L, Latini R, et al. Valsartan benefits left ventricular structure and function in heart failure: VaL-HeFT echocardiographic study. J Am Coll Cardiol 2002;40:970–5.

[49] Doughty RN, Whalley GA, Gamble G, et al. Left ventricular remodeling with carvedilol in patients with congestive heart failure due to ischemic heart disease. Australia-New Zealand Heart Failure Research Collaborative Group. J Am Coll Cardiol 1997;29:1060–6.

[50] Doughty RN, Whalley GA, Walsh HA, et al. Effects of carvedilol on left ventricular remodeling after acute myocardial infarction: the CAPRICORN Echo Substudy. Circulation 2004;109:201–6.

[51] Sliwa K, Norton GR, Kone N, et al. Impact of initiating carvedilol before angiotensin converting enzyme inhibitor therapy on cardiac function in newly diagnosed heart failure. J Am Coll Cardiol 2004;44:1825–30.

[52] Remme WJ, on behalf of the CARMEN Steering Committee and Investigators. The Carvedilol and

ACE-Inhibitor Remodelling Mild Heart Failure EvaluatioN trial (CARMEN)—rationale and design. Cardiovasc Drugs Ther 2001;15:69–77.

[53] Remme WJ, Riegger G, Hildebrandt P, et al, on behalf of the CARMEN investigators. The benefits of early combination treatment of carvedilol and an ACE-inhibitor in mild heart failure and left ventricular systolic dysfunction. The Carvedilol and Ace-inhibitor Remodelling Mild heart failure EvaluatioN trial (CARMEN). Cardiovasc Drugs Ther 2004;18:57–66.

[54] Willenheimer R, Erdmann E, Follath F, et al, on behalf of the CIBIS III investigators. Comparison of treatment initiation with bisoprolol versus enalapril in chronic heart failure patients: rationale and design of CIBIS-III. Eur J Heart Fail 2004;6:493–500.

[55] Willenheimer R, van Veldhuisen DJ, Silke B, et al, on behalf of the CIBIS III investigators. Effect on survival and hospitalization of initiating treatment for chronic heart failure with bisoprolol followed by enalapril, as compared with the opposite sequence. Results of the Randomized Cardiac Insufficiency Bisoprolol study (CIBIS) III. Circulation 2005;112:2426–35.

[56] Dickstein K. Clinical trials update from the European Society of Cardiology meeting 2005: CIBIS III. Response to correspondence from R. Willenheimer et al. Eur J Heart Fail 2006;8:221–2.

[57] Hall SA, Cigarro CG, Marcoux L, et al. Time course of improvement of left ventricular function, mass and geometry in patients with congestive heart failure treated with beta-adrenergic blockade. J Am Coll Cardiol 1995;25:1154–61.

[58] Remme WJ, Soler-Soler J, Ryden L. on behalf of the CARMEN investigators. Replacement of angiotensin converting enzyme inhibition by carvedilol results in long-term reversed left ventricular remodelling in mild heart failure and is well tolerated: Results of the CARMEN study. J Am Coll Cardiol 2003;41(suppl A):205A.

[59] Remme WJ, Riegger G, Ryden L, et al. Does baseline heart rate determine the effect of carvedilol on ventricular remodeling in heart failure? Results of the CARMEN trial. Eur Heart J 2003;24(abstract supplement):711.

CARDIOLOGY
CLINICS

Cardiol Clin 25 (2007) 595–603

Biventricular Pacing and Defibrillator Use in Chronic Heart Failure

David A. Cesario, MD, PhD[a], Jonathan W. Turner, MD[a],
G. William Dec, MD[b],*

[a]David Geffen School of Medicine at UCLA, Los Angeles, CA, USA
[b]Massachusetts General Hospital, Boston, MA, USA

Over the past 40 years, advances in our understanding of the pathophysiology and treatment of heart failure have led to significant improvements in survival and quality of life among patients affected by this disease [1–4]. Despite these advances, sudden cardiac death and progressive heart failure continue to present severe problems for heart failure patients and remain the major causes of mortality in this patient population [5]. Unfortunately, antiarrhythmic drugs have failed to reduce mortality rates among heart failure patients [6,7]. Recently, implantable cardioverter defibrillators (ICDs) and cardiac resynchronization therapy (CRT) have had major impacts on the treatment of heart failure in the United States. The use of ICDs, in addition to standard medical therapy, has resulted in significant survival benefits among survivors of ventricular fibrillation or sustained ventricular tachycardia [8–10]. However, the rates of successful resuscitation of out-of-hospital cardiac arrest patients remain woefully low [11], resulting in the application of ICD therapy for primary prevention in certain patients at high risk for cardiac arrest. Disturbances in electrical conduction, or electrical dyssynchrony, result in inefficient mechanical contraction of the ventricle and are an important cause of chronic left ventricular systolic dysfunction. Cardiac resynchronization therapy (CRT) is acutely associated with improved contractility, decreased mitral regurgitation, and lowered left ventricular filling pressures. CRT alone or when combined with defibrillation (CRTD), has been demonstrated to have major beneficial effects on the overall morbidity and mortality of heart failure [12,13]. This review will focus on the available guidelines and major clinical trial results to help guide the practicing clinician on the appropriate use of these implantable devices in patients with heart failure as a result of systolic dysfunction.

ICDs in survivors of prior cardiac arrest

Sudden cardiac death remains an important cause of mortality in the United States, accounting for 200,000 to 450,000 deaths annually and comprising more than half of all cardiovascular mortalities [14–16]. Patients who have been successfully resuscitated from cardiac arrest remain at high risk of developing future life-threatening ventricular arrhythmias [14,17–20]. ICD therapy remains the only evidence-based therapeutic strategy for survivors of life-threatening ventricular arrhythmic events [21]. Table 1 lists the American College of Cardiology/American Heart Association/North American Society for Pacing and Electrophysiology (ACC/AHA/NASPE) 2002 guidelines for ICD implantation [22]. It is readily apparent that the class I indications for ICDs are heavily based on the strong evidence for defibrillator therapy in survivors of cardiac arrest. Several prospective, controlled secondary prevention studies specifically examined the use of ICDs in this population. The Antiarrhythmics Versus Implantable Defibrillators (AVID) trial [9]

---

* Corresponding author.
  E-mail address: gdec@partners.org (G.W. Dec).

Table 1
American College of Cardiology/American Heart Association/North American Society for Pacing and Electrophysiology (ACC/AHA/NASPE) 2002 Guidelines for Implantable Cardioverter-Defibrillators

Class I indications	Level of evidence
Cardiac arrest due to VT or VF, not due to a transient/reversible cause.	A
Spontaneous sustained VT in patients with structural heart disease	B
Syncope of undetermined origin in patients with clinically relevant, hemodynamically significant VT or VF induced at EPS and refractory to drug therapy	B
Nonsustained VT in patients with CAD, prior MI, and inducible VT at EPS that is not suppressed by class I antiarrhythmic drugs.	A
Class IIa Indications	
Patients with left ventricular ejection fraction <30%, at least 1 month post-MI and 3 months post-CABG	B
Class IIb Indications	
Cardiac arrest presumed to be due to VF when EPS is precluded by other medical conditions.	C
Severe symptoms (eg, syncope) attributed to VT in patients awaiting cardiac transplantation.	C
Familial or inherited conditions with a high risk of life-threatening VT such as LQTS or HCM.	B
Nonsustained VT with CAD, prior MI, LV dysfunction, and inducible VT or VF at EPS.	B
Recurrent syncope of undetermined etiology in the presence of LV dysfunction and inducible VT at EPS when other causes of syncope have been excluded.	C
Syncope in patients with advanced structural heart disease in which thorough invasive and noninvasive testing has not shown a cause	C

Abbreviations: CABG, coronary artery bypass grafting; CAD, coronary artery disease; EPS, electrophysiologic study; HCM, hypertrophic cardiomyopathy; LQTS, long QT syndrome; LV, left ventricular; MI, myocardial infarction; NYHA, New York Heart Association; VF, ventricular fibrillation; VT, ventricular tachycardia.

Data from Gregoratos G, Abrams J, Epstein AE, et al. ACC/AHA/NASPE 2002 guideline update for implantation of cardiac pacemakers and antiarrhythmia devices: summary article. A report of the American College of Cardiology/American Heart Association Task Force on Practice Guidelines (ACC/AHA/NASPE Committee to Update the 1998 Pacemaker Guidelines). Circulation 2002;106(16):2145–61; and Cesario DA, Dec GW. Implantable cardioverter-defibrillator therapy in clinical practice. J Am Coll Cardiol 2006;47(8):1507–17.

enrolled 1016 patients who either survived ventricular fibrillation (VF) arrest, had a history of syncope due to sustained ventricular tachycardia (VT) requiring cardioversion, or had depressed left ventricular ejection fraction (LVEF) (<40%) and severe cardiac symptoms suggestive of malignant arrhythmias. Patients in the AVID trial were randomized to receive either ICD therapy or treatment with a class III antiarrhythmic drug, primarily amiodarone, at empirically determined doses. Over a mean follow-up period of 18.2 months, patients in the ICD group were found to have statistically significant relative risk reductions in overall mortality at 1, 2, and 3 years of follow-up (P < .02) [9]. Similar patient populations were enrolled in the underpowered Canadian Implantable Defibrillator Study (CIDS) [10] and Cardiac Arrest Study Hamburg (CASH) [8] trials, which trended toward mortality reduction, but did not reach statistical significance among

ICD recipients. However, a meta-analysis of pooled data from the AVID, CIDS, and CASH trials clearly demonstrated a 28% relative-risk reduction in total mortality with the greatest benefit observed in patients with LVEF of 20% to 34% [23]. Based on the results of these 3 landmark trials, the ACC/AHA/NASPE guidelines give a class I recommendation for ICD implantation in survivors of cardiac arrest as a result of VT or VF not due to reversible or transient causes such as myocardial ischemia.

ICDs for primary prevention of sudden death in ischemic cardiomyopathy

Patients with coronary artery disease (CAD) and left ventricular dysfunction are at high risk for lethal ventricular arrhythmias and the probability of sudden cardiac death increases in a nearly exponential manner as left ejection fraction falls below 30% [11,24,25]. Several randomized clinical trials have evaluated primary prevention ICD therapy among patients with impaired left ventricular systolic function due to underlying ischemic heart disease. The first Multicenter Automatic Defibrillator Implantation Trial (MADIT-I) demonstrated the superiority of ICDs to conventional medical therapy in patients with a history of myocardial infarction (MI) and LVEF of 35% or less, a history of spontaneous nonsustained VT, and inducible VT during electrophysiologic (EP) testing that was not suppressed during intravenous procainamide infusion [26]. The Multicenter Unsustained Tachycardia Trial (MUSTT) evaluated the efficacy of EP-guided antiarrhythmic therapy versus conventional medical therapy in patients with inducible VT on EP testing [6]. Patients enrolled in this trial could receive an ICD without randomization if one or more drug trials showed inadequate ventricular arrhythmia suppression. After 5 years of follow-up, all-cause mortality was significantly reduced in patients receiving ICD therapy ($P < .001$) compared with both conventional medical therapy and EP-guided antiarrhythmic therapy [6]. Ultimately, the conclusions drawn from MADIT-I and MUSTT culminated in the ACC/AHA/NASPE guidelines issuing a class I indication for ICD implantation in patients with ischemic cardiomyopathy who have a history of nonsustained VT and prior MI with inducible VF or sustained VT at EP study that is refractory to Class I antiarrhythmic medications.

The broader utility of ICDs in primary prevention was not fully appreciated until the MADIT investigators published a second study (MADIT-II) demonstrating the efficacy of prophylactic ICD implantation in patients with a history of prior MI and LVEF of 30% or less even without evidence for an inducible ventricular arrhythmia [27]. In MADIT-II, during an average follow-up of 20 months, ICD therapy resulted in a 5.6% absolute risk reduction compared with standard medical therapy ($P = .016$) [27]. It should be noted however, that 2 ICD trials have failed to demonstrate a survival benefit for defibrillators over standard medical therapy in patients with CAD and left ventricular dysfunction. The Coronary Artery Bypass Graft Trial (CABG Patch) was one such study that randomized patients with a LVEF less than 36% already scheduled for elective coronary revascularization surgery to undergo ICD implantation versus no

ICD (control group) at the time of their coronary artery bypass graft surgery [28]. In this trial, there was essentially no change in survival between patients receiving ICDs versus controls. The relative risk ratio for death in ICD patients was 1.07 (95% confidence interval, 0.81 to 1.42; P = not significant). However, it should be noted that most deaths in the ICD group in this trial occurred in the perioperative period and that 10% of the control group eventually crossed over to receive ICD therapy during the trial [28]. The Defibrillator in Acute Myocardial Infarction Trial (DINAMIT) also showed no mortality reduction among patients with a LVEF of 35% or less and impaired cardiac autonomic function (decreased heart rate variability or elevated average heart rate as determined by 24-hour ambulatory monitoring) treated with prophylactic ICD implantation during the early post-MI period (6 to 40 days after MI) [29]. Given the data represented by these trials, current guidelines recommend ICD implantation in patients who are at least 1 month post-MI with a LVEF 30% or less and at least 3 months postpercutaneous coronary intervention or CABG.

Current guidelines for prophylactic ICD implantation suffer from the fact that the use of LVEF alone for identification of patients at high or low risk for sudden cardiac death is limited by its low specificity. Findings in the Sudden Cardiac Death in Heart Failure Trial (SCD-HeFT) indicate that 81% of treated patients receive no benefit from ICD therapy at 5-year follow-up [7]. The need for more accurate risk stratification strategies beyond depressed LVEF and New York Heart Association (NYHA) functional classification to more precisely identify which heart failure patients are most (and least) likely to benefit from ICD therapy is great. Retrospective posthoc analyses from the MADIT-II trial suggest that patients with preserved systolic and diastolic blood pressure may derive little or no benefit from ICD implantation [30]. A normal microvolt T-wave alternans study also appears useful for identifying low-risk patients with ischemic left ventricular dysfunction based on a limited number of studies [31].

ICDs for primary prevention in nonischemic cardiomyopathy

Early trials that investigated primary prevention of sudden cardiac death in patients with nonischemic cardiomyopathy gave mixed results. However, several more recent trials have suggested a beneficial role for ICD therapy in this patient population. The Cardiomyopathy Trial (CAT) enrolled 104 patients with nonischemic dilated cardiomyopathy of recent onset (<9 months) and an LVEF of 30% or less to receive either an ICD or conventional medical therapy [32]. This trial was terminated early because all-cause mortality at 1-year follow-up did not reach the expected 30% in the control group. However, analysis of the existing data revealed no significant difference in survival between patients receiving ICDs versus control patients in this underpowered trial [32]. Additionally, the Amiodarone Versus Implantable Cardioverter Defibrillator Trial (AMIOVIRT) showed no survival benefits with ICD therapy over amiodarone in patients with nonischemic dilated cardiomyopathy, LVEF 35% or less, and asymptomatic nonsustained ventricular tachycardia [33]. Several studies have confirmed the prognostic importance of syncope in patients with nonischemic cardiomyopathy and reduced LVEF, suggesting a potential survival benefit with ICD therapy in this specific patient population [34,35].

The Defibrillators in Non-Ischemic Cardiomyopathy Treatment Evaluation (DEFINITE) trial randomized patients with nonischemic dilated cardiomyopathy, LVEF less than 36%, and more than 10 premature ventricular complexes per hour or nonsustained ventricular tachycardia on 24-hour ambulatory monitoring to receive standard medical therapy alone, or in combination with an ICD [36]. ICD therapy resulted in a trend toward improved overall survival at 24 months but failed to reach statistical significance ($P = .08$); however, there was a marked reduction in the secondary end point, risk of sudden death from arrhythmias, in patients receiving an ICD [36]. The SCD-HeFT enrolled patients with LVEF less than 35%, ischemic (52%) or nonischemic (48%) cardiomyopathy, and NYHA functional class II (70%) or III (30%) heart failure symptoms to receive conventional medical therapy alone, or in combination with either amiodarone or an ICD [7]. Over a median follow-up of 45.5 months, SCD-HeFT demonstrated a significant survival benefit in patients receiving ICDs, regardless of etiology (nonischemic and ischemic), while amiodarone therapy failed to improve survival [7]. These recent trials suggest that ICDs provide a survival benefit for patients with nonischemic dilated cardiomyopathy of greater than 9 months' duration, a LVEF 35% or less, and NYHA Class II or III heart failure as is reflected in the Centers for Medicare and Medicaid Services guidelines for implantation of ICDs (Box 1).

The timing of ICD implantation in patients with new-onset dilated cardiomyopathy remains controversial. Sufficient time should elapse to ensure that significant recovery of left ventricular systolic function does not occur. Yet, the risk of sudden cardiac death persists during each month that left ventricular ejection fraction remains depressed. Retrospective data from the DEFINITE trial demonstrate the same benefit for patients with new-onset dilated cardiomyopathy (<3 months) compared with patients who have more long-standing disease [37]. The current recommendation of waiting 9 months for ICD implantation in patients with new-onset nonischemic cardiomyopathies may not be applicable to all subgroups of patients and will require further study.

Cardiac resynchronization therapy in heart failure

Ventricular dyssynchrony is a state of uncoordinated electrical activation of the heart resulting in different portions of the ventricle contracting at different times. This results in a highly inefficient contractile state as opposed to the normal heart in which all segments contract nearly simultaneously [38]. Evidence of ventricular dyssynchrony can be seen on the surface ECG as a prolongation of the QRS duration, most often with a left bundle branch block pattern. QRS prolongation has been associated with diminished cardiac function, more advanced heart failure symptoms, and worsened survival [39–41]. Approximately 30% of patients with NYHA class II through IV heart failure symptoms will also have ventricular dyssynchrony as defined by significant QRS prolongation. Cardiac resynchronization therapy (CRT) uses a left ventricular lead positioned on the lateral wall of the left ventricle either endovascularly via the coronary sinus or epicardially via direct surgical placement on the left ventricle. Placement of the additional lead on the lateral wall of the left ventricle ensures near simultaneous stimulation of both ventricles. Acutely, CRT has been associated with improved contractility, decreased mitral regurgitation, and decreased left ventricular filling pressures. Successful biventricular pacing typically results in an improvement in symptoms by one NYHA functional class and at

least 20% improvement in scores on the Minnesota Living with Heart Failure Questionnaire.

Proper patient selection for CRT remains an
important issue. Published studies suggest that
only 70% of heart failure patients receiving
a biventricular device experience a measurable
clinical improvement from CRT. Biventricular
pacing often does not benefit patients with left
ventricular ejection fractions of more than 40%,
probably because heart failure in such patients is
largely due to diastolic dysfunction. Ambulatory
patients with severe (NYHA functional class III
or IV) symptoms despite optimized medical therapy (including a diuretic regimen, an angiotensin-
converting enzyme inhibitor, and a beta-blocker,
with or without an aldosterone antagonist) appear
to derive the greatest benefit from CRT. Within
this population, most clinical trials to date have
focused on patients in normal sinus rhythm with
a QRS duration more than 130 ms; however, it is
increasingly evident that QRS duration alone is
a crude measure for evaluating ventricular dyssynchrony. Recent studies have shown a surprisingly poor correlation between QRS duration on
the surface ECG and the extent of mechanical
dyssynchrony (r correlation <0.30) [42]. Newer
approaches that show promise in predicting clinical response to cardiac resynchronization include
contrast-enhanced magnetic resonance imaging
to assess the amount of fixed scarring, tissue
Doppler imaging, and speckle-tracking radial
strain imaging [43,44]. Table 2 highlights the
most recent Heart Failure Society of America's
guidelines for CRT [45].

Over the past several years numerous trials
have shown the benefits of CRT in the chronic
heart failure population. The Multisite Stimulation in Cardiomyopathies (MUSTIC) trial enrolled patients with NYHA class III heart failure
symptoms, sinus rhythm and QRS duration more
than 150 ms in a single-blind, randomized, controlled cross-over fashion, to receive 3 months of
biventricular pacing and 3 months of inactive
pacing (VVI backup at 40 beats/min) [46]. During
the active CRT period, patients experienced a significant improvement in 6-minute walk distance
(+30 m or more) [46]. The Multicenter InSync
Randomized Clinical Evaluation (MIRACLE)
trial similarly showed that cardiac resynchronization improved 6-minute walk distance in patients
with moderate to severe heart failure compared
with controls receiving standard medical therapy
[47]. Furthermore, the CONTAK-CD, InSync
ICD [48], and MIRACLE [47] trials demonstrated

Table 2
Heart Failure Society of America: device treatment guidelines for CRT in HF

Guideline	Level of evidence
Persistent moderate to severe HF (NYHA class III) despite optimal medical therapy with sinus rhythm, widened QRS ($\geq$ 120 ms), severe LV systolic dysfunction (LVEF $\leq$ 35%) and LV dilatation ($>$5.5 cm)	A
Selected ambulatory NYHA class IV patients	B
Biventricular pacing therapy is NOT recommended in patients who are asymptomatic or have mild HF symptoms	C

Abbreviations: CRT, cardiac resynchronization therapy; HF, heart failure; LV, left ventricular; LVEF, left ventricular ejection fraction; ms, milliseconds; NYHA, New York Heart Association.
Data from Adams KF, Lindenfeld J, Arnold JM, et al. Executive Summary: HFSA 2006 Comprehensive Heart Failure Practice Guidelines. J Cardiac Failure 2006;12:10–38.

a reduction in heart failure hospitalizations in patients receiving CRT.

The Comparison of Medical Therapy, Pacing and Defibrillators in Chronic Heart Failure (COMPANION) trial was the first large-scale prospective trial to directly examine the effects of CRT on all-cause mortality [12]. Patients with either ischemic or non-ischemic cardiomyopathy, left ventricular ejection fractions of 35% or less, and NYHA functional class III or IV symptoms were randomized to receive optimal medical therapy alone, biventricular pacing, or biventricular pacing combined with ICD. This trial showed a trend toward reduction in all-cause mortality in patients receiving CRT (14.4% absolute mortality reduction for biventricular pacing versus 19% for optimal medical therapy alone). Furthermore, patients receiving biventricular pacing plus a defibrillator had a statistically significant reduction in all-cause mortality (absolute mortality, 11%; $P < .01$) [12]. Importantly, in a cohort of patients with advanced symptoms (n = 213), cardiac resynchronization either with or without an ICD was shown to improve all-cause mortality and hospitalization rates for ambulatory NYHA class IV patients with a strong trend toward improved overall mortality in this population [49]. The Cardiac Resynchronization-Heart Failure (CARE-HF) study solidified the mortality benefits of CRT in patients with advanced symptomatic heart failure (NYHA functional class III or IV) caused by left ventricular systolic dysfunction with evidence of ventricular dyssynchrony [13]. In CARE-HF, CRT resulted in significant improvements over standard medical therapy in the composite primary end point of death from any cause or unplanned hospitalization for a major cardiovascular event. Furthermore, CRT resulted

in significant reductions in the interventricular mechanical delay, end-systolic volume index, and mitral regurgitant jet area when compared with medical therapy in the CARE-HF population [13]. Based on these trials, current practice guidelines support the use of biventricular pacing in patients with advanced (NYHA functional class III or IV) heart failure symptoms due to either ischemic or nonischemic cardiomyopathy when sinus rhythm, QRS prolongation ($>$120 ms), left ventricular enlargement (LV end-diastolic dimension $>$55 mm), and left ventricular systolic dysfunction (LVEF $\leq$ 35%) also exist [50]. However, indications for CRT may soon expand as small studies have suggested this treatment may improve symptoms and outcomes for patients with normal or mildly prolonged QRS duration ($<$120 msec) and those with chronic atrial fibrillation [51–54].

The Dual Chamber and VVI Implantable Defibrillator (DAVID) trial suggested that it may be useful to revise standard VVI or DDD pacemakers to CRT devices in patients with left ventricular dysfunction and chronic heart failure symptoms [55]. In the DAVID study, patients with ICDs had their devices programmed with either DDD rate-responsive pacing (set at 70 beats/min) or VVI pacing (set at 40 beats/min). Patients with DDD rate-responsive pacing had a trend toward increased mortality and heart failure hospitalizations when compared with the VVI pacing cohort [55]. Similar results were observed in the MADIT-II cohort randomized to ICD therapy who showed a high frequency of right ventricular pacing. These findings suggest that unnecessary right ventricular apical pacing may induce ventricular dyssynchrony and should be avoided, when possible, in patients with severe systolic dysfunction.

However, it should be pointed out that both studies were retrospective post hoc analyses and should thus be interpreted with some caution. Prospective controlled trials are still necessary to determine whether heart failure patients who require frequent ventricular pacing from a standard pacemaker or ICD would benefit from an upgrade to a biventricular device. Finally, the benefits of CRT in patients with asymptomatic left ventricular dysfunction or mild heart failure (NYHA functional class I or II) remain unclear and further clinical trials are underway to establish the possible utility of CRT in these patient populations.

Heart failure subsets in which ICD therapy is not clinically indicated

ICD therapy should not be used for patients with advanced heart failure symptoms (NYHA class IV) that remain refractory to optimal medical therapy and for whom cardiac transplantation is not an option. However, a select number of these patients may still be candidates for CRT with ICD backup capability. Previous studies have shown negligible survival benefits with ICD therapy in these patients; most die of progressive pump failure [56]. Furthermore, ICD therapy is contraindicated in the presence of medically intractable ventricular tachycardia or ventricular fibrillation, in patients with terminal illnesses and life expectancies of less than 6 months, and significant psychiatric illnesses that may be aggravated by device implantation or may preclude regular follow-up [22]. ICD implantation is also not recommended in patients with ventricular tachyarrhythmias due to a transient or reversible disorder (eg, electrolyte imbalance or drugs) when correction of the disorder is considered feasible and likely to substantially reduce the risk of recurrent ventricular arrhythmias [22]. Finally, ICD implantation remains unproven for patients with substantially impaired systolic function and coronary artery disease who lack evidence of sustained or nonsustained ventricular tachycardia and are scheduled to undergo coronary revascularization.

Summary

Since the 1970s, when the ICD was initially developed, there have been multiple clinical trials documenting the dramatic survival benefits of ICD therapy in certain high-risk subsets of heart failure patients. Over the past decade, CRT has also emerged as an important therapy in the treatment of chronic heart failure in carefully selected patients with ongoing symptoms despite optimized pharmacological therapy. ICDs should be considered first-line therapy for survivors of life-threatening ventricular arrhythmic events. Additionally, specific subsets of patients with both ischemic and nonischemic dilated cardiomyopathy appear to have a survival benefit from primary ICD therapy. Finally, CRT has also been clearly demonstrated to result in substantial symptomatic improvements and survival benefits in a subgroup of chronic heart failure patients. CRT should be considered in all patients undergoing ICD implantation who have evidence of ventricular dyssynchrony.

References

[1] Franciosa JA, Limas CJ, Guiha NH, et al. Improved left ventricular function during nitroprusside infusion in acute myocardial infarction. Lancet 1972; 1(7752):650–4.

[2] Pfeffer MA, Braunwald E, Moye LA, et al. Effect of captopril on mortality and morbidity in patients with left ventricular dysfunction after myocardial infarction. Results of the survival and ventricular enlargement trial. The SAVE Investigators. N Engl J Med 1992;327(10):669–77.

[3] Pitt B, Zannad F, Remme WJ, et al. The effect of spironolactone on morbidity and mortality in patients with severe heart failure. Randomized Aldactone Evaluation Study Investigators. N Engl J Med 1999;341(10):709–17.

[4] Packer M, Coats AJ, Fowler MB, et al. Effect of carvedilol on survival in severe chronic heart failure. N Engl J Med 2001;344(22):1651–8.

[5] Kadish A, Mehra M. Heart failure devices: implantable cardioverter-defibrillators and biventricular pacing therapy. Circulation 2005;111(24):3327–35.

[6] Buxton AE, Lee KL, Fisher JD, et al. A randomized study of the prevention of sudden death in patients with coronary artery disease. Multicenter Unsustained Tachycardia Trial Investigators. N Engl J Med 1999;341(25):1882–90.

[7] Bardy GH, Lee KL, Mark DB, et al. Amiodarone or an implantable cardioverter-defibrillator for congestive heart failure. N Engl J Med 2005;352(3):225–37.

[8] Siebels J, Cappato R, Ruppel R, et al. Preliminary results of the Cardiac Arrest Study Hamburg (CASH). CASH Investigators. Am J Cardiol 1993; 72(16):109F–13F.

[9] A comparison of antiarrhythmic-drug therapy with implantable defibrillators in patients resuscitated from near-fatal ventricular arrhythmias. The Antiarrhythmics versus Implantable Defibrillators

(AVID) Investigators. N Engl J Med 1997;337(22):1576–83.

[10] Connolly SJ, Gent M, Roberts RS, et al. Canadian implantable defibrillator study (CIDS): a randomized trial of the implantable cardioverter defibrillator against amiodarone. Circulation 2000;101(11):1297–302.

[11] Huikuri HV, Castellanos A, Myerburg RJ. Sudden death due to cardiac arrhythmias. N Engl J Med 2001;345(20):1473–82.

[12] Bristow MR, Saxon LA, Boehmer J, et al. Cardiac-resynchronization therapy with or without an implantable defibrillator in advanced chronic heart failure. N Engl J Med 2004;350(21):2140–50.

[13] Cleland JG, Daubert JC, Erdmann E, et al. The effect of cardiac resynchronization on morbidity and mortality in heart failure. N Engl J Med 2005;352(15):1539–49.

[14] Myerburg RJ, Kessler KM, Castellanos A. Sudden cardiac death: epidemiology, transient risk, and intervention assessment. Ann Intern Med 1993;119(12):1187–97.

[15] Escobedo LG, Zack MM. Comparison of sudden and nonsudden coronary deaths in the United States. Circulation 1996;93(11):2033–6.

[16] Zheng ZJ, Croft JB, Giles WH, et al. Sudden cardiac death in the United States, 1989 to 1998. Circulation 2001;104(18):2158–63.

[17] Baum RS, Alvarez H 3rd, Cobb LA. Survival after resuscitation from out-of-hospital ventricular fibrillation. Circulation 1974;50(6):1231–5.

[18] Eisenberg MS, Hallstrom A, Bergner L. Long-term survival after out-of-hospital cardiac arrest. N Engl J Med 1982;306(22):1340–3.

[19] Goldstein S, Landis JR, Leighton R, et al. Predictive survival models for resuscitated victims of out-of-hospital cardiac arrest with coronary heart disease. Circulation 1985;71(5):873–80.

[20] Myerburg RJ, Kessler KM, Estes D, et al. Long-term survival after prehospital cardiac arrest: analysis of outcome during an 8 year study. Circulation 1984;70(4):538–46.

[21] Cesario DA, Dec GW. Implantable cardioverter-defibrillator therapy in clinical practice. J Am Coll Cardiol 2006;47(8):1507–17.

[22] Gregoratos G, Abrams J, Epstein AE, et al. ACC/AHA/NASPE 2002 guideline update for implantation of cardiac pacemakers and antiarrhythmia devices: summary article. A report of the American College of Cardiology/American Heart Association Task Force on Practice Guidelines (ACC/AHA/NASPE Committee to Update the 1998 Pacemaker Guidelines). Circulation 2002;106(16):2145–61.

[23] Oseroff O, Retyk E, Bochoeyer A. Subanalyses of secondary prevention implantable cardioverter-defibrillator trials: antiarrhythmics versus implantable defibrillators (AVID), Canadian Implantable Defibrillator Study (CIDS), and Cardiac Arrest Study Hamburg (CASH). Curr Opin Cardiol 2004;19(1):26–30.

[24] Priori SG, Aliot E, Blomstrom-Lundqvist C, et al. Task Force on sudden cardiac death of the European Society of Cardiology. Eur Heart J 2001;22(16):1374–450.

[25] Rouleau JL, Talajic M, Sussex B, et al. Myocardial infarction patients in the 1990s—their risk factors, stratification and survival in Canada: the Canadian Assessment of Myocardial Infarction (CAMI) Study. J Am Coll Cardiol 1996;27(5):1119–27.

[26] Moss AJ, Hall WJ, Cannon DS, et al. Improved survival with an implanted defibrillator in patients with coronary disease at high risk for ventricular arrhythmia. Multicenter Automatic Defibrillator Implantation Trial Investigators. N Engl J Med 1996;335(26):1933–40.

[27] Moss AJ, Zareba W, Hall WJ, et al. Prophylactic implantation of a defibrillator in patients with myocardial infarction and reduced ejection fraction. N Engl J Med 2002;346(12):877–83.

[28] Bigger JT Jr. Prophylactic use of implanted cardiac defibrillators in patients at high risk for ventricular arrhythmias after coronary-artery bypass graft surgery. Coronary Artery Bypass Graft (CABG) Patch Trial Investigators. N Engl J Med 1997;337(22):1569–75.

[29] Hohnloser SH, Kuck KH, Dorian P, et al. Prophylactic use of an implantable cardioverter-defibrillator after acute myocardial infarction. N Engl J Med 2004;351(24):2481–8.

[30] Goldenberg I, Moss AJ, McNitt S, et al. Inverse relationship of blood pressure levels to sudden cardiac mortality and benefit of the implantable cardioverter-defibrillator in patients with ischemic left ventricular dysfunction. J Am Coll Cardiol 2007;49(13):1427–33.

[31] Chow T, Kereiakes DJ, Bartone C, et al. Microvolt T-wave alternans identifies patients with ischemic cardiomyopathy who benefit from implantable cardioverter-defibrillator therapy. J Am Coll Cardiol 2007;49(1):50–8.

[32] Bansch D, Antz M, Boczor S, et al. Primary prevention of sudden cardiac death in idiopathic dilated cardiomyopathy: the Cardiomyopathy Trial (CAT). Circulation 2002;105(12):1453–8.

[33] Strickberger SA, Hummel JD, Bartlett TG, et al. Amiodarone versus implantable cardioverter-defibrillator:randomized trial in patients with nonischemic dilated cardiomyopathy and asymptomatic nonsustained ventricular tachycardia—AMIOVIRT. J Am Coll Cardiol 2003;41(10):1707–12.

[34] Fonarow GC, Feliciano Z, Boyle NG, et al. Improved survival in patients with nonischemic advanced heart failure and syncope treated with an implantable cardioverter-defibrillator. Am J Cardiol 2000;85(8):981–5.

[35] Knight BP, Goyal R, Pelosi F, et al. Outcome of patients with nonischemic dilated cardiomyopathy and unexplained syncope treated with an implantable defibrillator. J Am Coll Cardiol 1999;33(7):1964–70.

[36] Kadish A, Dyer A, Daubert JP, et al. Prophylactic defibrillator implantation in patients with nonischemic dilated cardiomyopathy. N Engl J Med 2004; 350(21):2151–8.

[37] Kadish A, Schaechter A, Subacius H, et al. Patients with recently diagnosed nonischemic cardiomyopathy benefit from implantable cardioverter-defibrillators. J Am Coll Cardiol 2006;47(12):2477–82.

[38] Burkhardt JD, Wilkoff BL. Interventional electrophysiology and cardiac resynchronization therapy: delivering electrical therapies for heart failure. Circulation 2007;115(16):2208–20.

[39] Baldasseroni S, Opasich C, Gorini M, et al. Left bundle-branch block is associated with increased 1-year sudden and total mortality rate in 5517 outpatients with congestive heart failure: a report from the Italian network on congestive heart failure. Am Heart J 2002;143(3):398–405.

[40] Aaronson KD, Schwartz JS, Chen TM, et al. Development and prospective validation of a clinical index to predict survival in ambulatory patients referred for cardiac transplant evaluation. Circulation 1997; 95(12):2660–7.

[41] Shamim W, Francis DP, Yousufuddin M, et al. Intraventricular conduction delay: a prognostic marker in chronic heart failure. Int J Cardiol 1999; 70(2):171–8.

[42] Bax JJ, Bleeker GB, Marwick TH, et al. Left ventricular dyssynchrony predicts response and prognosis after cardiac resynchronization therapy. J Am Coll Cardiol 2004;44(9):1834–40.

[43] Breithardt OA, Breithardt G. Quest for the best candidate: how much imaging do we need before prescribing cardiac resynchronization therapy? Circulation 2006;113(7):926–8.

[44] Suffoletto MS, Dohi K, Cannesson M, et al. Novel speckle-tracking radial strain from routine black-and-white echocardiographic images to quantify dyssynchrony and predict response to cardiac resynchronization therapy. Circulation 2006; 113(7):960–8.

[45] Heart Failure Society Of America. HFSA 2006 Comprehensive Heart Failure Practice Guideline. J Card Fail 2006;12(1):E1–2.

[46] Cazeau S, Leclercq C, Lavergne T, et al. Effects of multisite biventricular pacing in patients with heart failure and intraventricular conduction delay. N Engl J Med 2001;344(12):873–80.

[47] Abraham WT, Fisher WG, Smith AL, et al. Cardiac resynchronization in chronic heart failure. N Engl J Med 2002;346(24):1845–53.

[48] Gras D, Leclercq C, Tang AS, et al. Cardiac resynchronization therapy in advanced heart failure the multicenter InSync clinical study. Eur J Heart Fail 2002;4(3):311–20.

[49] Lindenfeld J, Feldman AM, Saxon L, et al. Effects of cardiac resynchronization therapy with or without a defibrillator on survival and hospitalizations in patients with New York Heart Association class IV heart failure. Circulation 2007;115(2):204–12.

[50] Strickberger SA, Conti J, Daoud EG, et al. Patient selection for cardiac resynchronization therapy: from the Council on Clinical Cardiology Subcommittee on Electrocardiography and Arrhythmias and the Quality of Care and Outcomes Research Interdisciplinary Working Group, in collaboration with the Heart Rhythm Society. Circulation 2005; 111(16):2146–50.

[51] Abraham WT. Cardiac resynchronization therapy is important for all patients with congestive heart failure and ventricular dyssynchrony. Circulation 2006; 114(24):2692–8 [discussion: 2698].

[52] Bleeker GB, Holman ER, Steendijk P, et al. Cardiac resynchronization therapy in patients with a narrow QRS complex. J Am Coll Cardiol 2006;48(11): 2243–50.

[53] Yu CM, Chan YS, Zhang Q, et al. Benefits of cardiac resynchronization therapy for heart failure patients with narrow QRS complexes and coexisting systolic asynchrony by echocardiography. J Am Coll Cardiol 2006;48(11):2251–7.

[54] Delnoy PP, Ottervanger JP, Luttikhuis HO, et al. Comparison of usefulness of cardiac resynchronization therapy in patients with atrial fibrillation and heart failure versus patients with sinus rhythm and heart failure. Am J Cardiol 2007;99(9):1252–7.

[55] Wilkoff BL, Cook JR, Epstein AE, et al. Dual-chamber pacing or ventricular backup pacing in patients with an implantable defibrillator: the Dual Chamber and VVI Implantable Defibrillator (DAVID) Trial. JAMA 2002;288(24):3115–23.

[56] Sweeney MO, Ruskin JN, Garan H, et al. Influence of the implantable cardioverter/defibrillator on sudden death and total mortality in patients evaluated for cardiac transplantation. Circulation 1995; 92(11):3273–81.

ELSEVIER
SAUNDERS

Cardiol Clin 25 (2007) 605–610

CARDIOLOGY
CLINICS

Index

Note: Page numbers of article titles are in **boldface** type.

A

ACC. See *American College of Cardiology (ACC)*.

ACE inhibitor/angiotensin receptor blockers, beta-blockers vs, **581–594.** See also *Beta-blocker(s), ACE inhibitor/angiotensin receptor blockers vs.*

ACE inhibitors. See *Angiotensin-converting enzyme (ACE) inhibitor(s)*.

Acute heart failure syndrome (AHFS), management of, pharmacologic therapy in, **539–551**
 carperitide, 543
 catecholamines, 545–546
 clinical development of
  challenges in, 546–548
  drug comparator in, 547
  endpoints in, 547
  future perspectives in, 547–548
  study population in, 546–547
  therapeutic targets in, 546
  timing and dosing of intervention in, 547
  trial designs in, 546
 diuretics, 539–541
 inotropic therapy, 544–546
 levosimendan, 545–546
 natriuretic peptides, 542–543
 nitroglycerin, 541–542
 nitroprusside, 541–542
 phosphodiesterase inhibitors, 545
 vasodilator therapy–targeting abnormal loading, 541–544
 vasopressin receptor antagonists, 541

ADHERE database, 544

Age, as factor in heart failure, 487

AHA. See *American Heart Association (AHA)*.

AHFS. See *Acute heart failure syndrome (AHFS)*.

Aldosterone antagonists, in diabetic heart failure management, 532–533

Aliskiren Observation of Heart Failure Treatment trial, 579

ALLHAT. See *Antihypertensive and Lipid-lowering Treatment to Prevent Heart Attack Trial (ALLHAT)*.

American College of Cardiology (ACC), 497

American College of Cardiology/American Heart Association (ACC/AHA), in heart failure management, 517–518

American Heart Association (AHA), 497

Amiodarone Versus Implantable Cardioverter Defibrillator Trial (AMIOVIRT), 598

AMIOVIRT. See *Amiodarone Versus Implantable Cardioverter Defibrillator Trial (AMIOVIRT)*.

Angiotensin receptor blockers, in heart failure chronic, rationale for, 574–579
 diabetic, 532
 rationale for, 573–574

Angiotensin-converting enzyme (ACE) inhibitor(s)
 as first-line therapy in heart failure, 581–583
 in diabetic heart failure management, 532
 in heart failure prevention, 516

Angiotensin-converting enzyme (ACE) inhibitor/ angiotensin receptor blockers, beta-blockers vs., **581–594.** See also *Beta-blocker(s), ACE inhibitor/angiotensin receptor blockers vs..*

Anglo–Scandinavian Cardiac Outcomes Trial-Blood Pressure Lowering Arm study, 515

Anti-angiotensin therapy, **573–580**

Antihypertensive and Lipid-lowering Treatment to Prevent Heart Attack Trial (ALLHAT), 513

ARDS Clinical Trials Network, 567

ATLAS (Assessment of Treatment with Lisinopril and Survival) study, 524

Moving?

Make sure your subscription moves with you!

To notify us of your new address, find your **Clinics Account Number** (located on your mailing label above your name), and contact customer service at:

E-mail: elspcs@elsevier.com

800-654-2452 (subscribers in the U.S. & Canada)
407-345-4000 (subscribers outside of the U.S. & Canada)

Fax number: 407-363-9661

Elsevier Periodicals Customer Service
6277 Sea Harbor Drive
Orlando, FL 32887-4800

*To ensure uninterrupted delivery of your subscription, please notify us at least 4 weeks in advance of move.

ELSEVIER